The OTA's Guide to Writing SOAP Notes

The OTA's Guide to Writing SOAP Notes

Sherry Borcherding, MA, OTR/L
University of Missouri
Columbia, Missouri

Carol Kappel, COTA/L
St. Louis Community College
Kirkwood, Missouri

SLACK
INCORPORATED
an innovative information, education, and management company
6900 Grove Road • Thorofare, NJ 08086

The procedures and practices described in this book should be implemented in a manner consistent with the professional standards set for the circumstances that apply in each specific situation. Every effort has been made to confirm the accuracy of the information presented and to correctly relate generally accepted practices. The author, editor, and publisher cannot accept responsibility for errors or exclusions or for the outcome of the application of the material presented herein. There is no expressed or implied warranty of this book or information imparted by it.

The work SLACK publishes is peer reviewed. Prior to publication, recognized leaders in the field, educators, and clinicians provide important feedback on the concepts and content that we publish. We welcome feedback on this work.

Borcherding, Sherry
The OTA's guide to writing SOAP notes / Sherry Borcherding, Carol Kappel.
p. ; cm.
Includes bibliographical refernces and index.
ISBN 1-55642-551-1 (alk. paper)
1. Occupational therapy assistants. 2. Medical records. 3. Medical writing. I. Kappel, Carol. II. Title.
[DNLM: 1. Occupayional Therapy--methods. 2. Allied Health Personnel. 3. Documentation--methods. 4. Medical Records. WB 555 B726o 2002]
RM735.4.B673 2002
615.8'515--dc21 2002019372

Printed in the United States of America

Published by: SLACK Incorporated
6900 Grove Road
Thorofare, NJ 08086 USA
Telephone: 856-848-1000
Fax: 856-853-5991
www.slackbooks.com

Contact SLACK Incorporated for more information about other books in this field or about the availability of our books from distributors outside the United States.

Last digit is print number: 10 9 8 7 6 5 4 3 2 1

Dedication

This book is dedicated to all the OT and OTA students we have taught, who have taught us so much about documentation

Contents

Acknowledgments

Many people have contributed to the development of this manual. First, I would like to thank Diana Baldwin, director of Occupational Therapy at the University of Missouri, for her patience in teaching me how to teach. Without her nurturing and support, I might have taken another pathway entirely. Thanks to Fred Dittrich for moving me as gracefully and quickly into the "information age" as I could tolerate. Thanks to Sandy Matsuda for her editing contributions, and for her loving friendship and support. Thanks to Doris O'Hara for bequeathing me the basic course material 7 years ago; and to Charlet Quay, Stephanie Owings, David Lackey, Lynne White, and LeaAnn Brittain for filling in the gaps in my knowledge base. Thanks to Leanna Garrison for being the Format Goddess. Thanks to Lenore Ball, Theresa Lackey, Chris Nelson, Linda Eagle, and Randy Kilgore for their help and support. But most of all, I would like to thank the students who have taught me so much about documentation over the past 10 years.

Sherry Borcherding, MA, OTR/L

I would like to acknowledge Nancy Klein and Harriet Backhaus, who expressed confidence in my ability to undertake this work. Their professional knowledge and experience in occupational therapy has been a great resource for me. My appreciation also goes to Amy McShane, editorial diretor at SLACK Incorporated, who gave me the opportunity to participate in this project and never tired of providing answers to my questions. I would also like to thank Sandy Matsuda for "introducing me" to Sherry and to the idea of editing this book for OTAs. I also want to personally thank my family: Jenna, Mike, Becca, Paul, and Brighid for their encouragement and constant support. And to my husband, Dean, who served as sounding board, proofreader, and counselor—my deepest appreciation.

Carol Kappel, COTA/L

About the Authors

Sherry Borcherding, MA, OTR/L currently serves as a faculty member at University of Missouri at Columbia, a Research I University, where she has taught for 7 years. She teaches disability awareness, loss and grief, and a three-semester fieldwork sequence designed to develop critical thinking, clinical reasoning, and documentation skills. She has also taught clinical ethics, frames of reference, psychopathology, long term-care, and wellness. Two of her courses are designated as campus writing courses and one is credentialed for computer and information proficiency. Sherry is frequently invited to present on collaborative learning and peer review as teaching strategies. In addition, she was one of a small group of campus faculty initially selected to develop web-based courses.

Sherry graduated with honors from Texas Woman's University with a bachelor of science in occupational therapy and went on to complete her master's degree in special education at George Peabody College in Nashville, TN. Following her staff positions in rehabilitation, home health, and pediatrics, she assumed a number of management roles including chief occupational therapist at East Texas Treatment Center, director of Occupational Therapy at Mid-Missouri Mental Health Center, and director of Rehabilitation Services at Transitional Housing Agency. She has also planned, designed, and directed occupational therapy programs at Charles E. Still Hospital in Jefferson City, MO and at Charter Behavioral Health Center in Columbia, MO.

Besides teaching, Sherry consults on quality assurance issues for local behavioral health centers and has a private practice devoted to complementary and alternative therapies. She is certified in CranioSacral Therapy at the techniques level through Upledger Institute and is attuned as a Reiki master. For leisure, Sherry enjoys folk dance, music, and all kinds of three-dimensional art. Her pottery has appeared in three local shows over the past 4 years.

Carol Kappel, COTA/L works at St. Louis Community College at Meramec as adjunct faculty in the Occupational Therapy Assistant and Physical Therapy Assistant Programs. She received her applied science degree in OTA from this program in 1990, participating in the honors program and graduating with highest honors. Before teaching, Carol worked as a COTA in long-term care facilities with special interest in positioning interventions and fabricating customized positioning equipment. She is also a registered medical technologist (MT/ASCP) and has worked in hospital and research labs.

Along with her current teaching duties, Carol enjoys participating in several church activities, including choir and the "special needs ministry," which seeks to reduce barriers that may prevent those with disabilities from participating and serving in church functions and activities. Her leisure pursuits include painting with watercolors, figure-drawing in pastels, and gardening.

Chapter One

Documenting the Treatment Process in Occupational Therapy

Introduction

Professional documentation is an important part of what occupational therapy assistants (OTAs) do. To an inexperienced OTA, the task of writing a note in a patient's chart can seem more difficult than providing the patient's treatment in the first place. How do you communicate in writing all that you have observed during your treatments in an accurate and concise manner that is both readable and understandable to others? No wonder this can seem like such an intimidating part of your job.

Professional documentation is a skill, and like any skill, it can be learned. Learning a skill, whether it is downhill skiing, playing the violin, or composing a treatment note, requires two things of you: instruction on how to do it (what to put into each section of the note) and practice (with feedback on which parts are correct and which still need work). This manual is designed to get you started with both parts of the process. Information is provided on each part of the documentation process, and the worksheets are designed to let you practice each step as you learn it.

The format for writing SOAP notes provided in this manual is one that is reimbursable under both Medicare Part B and managed care. While all notes do not have to meet these requirements, the Medicare B and managed care standards are the most rigorous. If you learn to meet these standards you are not likely to be denied by any third party payer.

Current occupational therapy practice is in many ways determined by which services are reimbursable, and documentation of patient care is the vehicle by which that service is communicated. Many therapists were not taught how to write effective notes and had to learn it on the job. They have learned what works in their own situation, but may or may not be prepared to meet the requirements of other settings.

The *Standards for an Accredited Educational Program for the Occupational Therapy Assistant* (Accreditation Council for Occupational Therapy Education [ACOTE], 1999) states that accredited OTA programs must contain curriculum that will facilitate the development of documentation skills to "ensure accountability of service provision and ...meet standards for reimbursement of services. Documentation shall effectively communicate the need and rationale for occupational therapy services" (ACOTE, 1999, Section B3.4). This manual will provide you with a mechanism for becoming competent in documentation skills.

The content of this manual reflects the scope of our practice and emphasizes the basis of our services, i.e., the use of occupation through occupational performance. Material from the following official documents of the American Occupational Therapy Association (AOTA) has been incorporated:

- *Elements of Clinical Documentation* (Thomson & Foto, 1995)
- *Occupational Therapy Code of Ethics* (AOTA, 2000)
- *Occupational Therapy Roles* (AOTA Intercommission Council, 1993)
- *Service Delivery in Occupational Therapy* (AOTA, 1995)
- *Standards of Practice for Occupational Therapy* (AOTA, 1998)
- *Uniform Terminology for Occupational Therapy, Third Edition* (AOTA Termilology Task Force, 1994)
- *The Guide to Occupational Therapy Practice* (Moyers, 1999)

Although OTAs write in more than one format, this manual presents a systematic approach to writing one form of documentation, the SOAP note. The manual is designed as a teaching tool and is most effective if used as a workbook, reading the information in each section, completing each exercise, and then checking your answers against the suggested answers. The original material presented in this book grew out of a course on documentation that has been taught for 10 years to occupational therapy students at the University of Missouri at Columbia. The book in its present form has been edited to make the content more specific to the documentation provided by OTAs in fulfilling their function in the clinical setting.

The information in this manual has been arranged in the order that it is most easily learned, with the more straightforward concepts being offered first. More complex concepts build on these as clinical reasoning is developed. *Chapter Two: The Medical Record* provides an introduction to the medical record—its function, uses, and history. The history of the SOAP note is included, along with the mechanics of writing in the record. Also included in Chapter Two is a list of standard abbreviations to be used in completing the exercises in the manual.

The next four chapters teach the four sections of the SOAP format (Subjective, Objective, Assessment, and Plan) that has been introduced and explained in Chapter Two. Multiple examples are presented for each section, and worksheets are provided for practice. It is difficult to learn documentation without observing treatment sessions upon which to base the notes, and it is assumed that you will have access to a treatment setting in which to document.

Chapter Seven: Goals and Interventions develops the subject of writing goals that are functional, measurable, and observable. In this same chapter we will discuss the ways that interventions differ from goals and provide some opportunities to practice writing both.

Chapter Eight: Documenting Different Stages of Treatment discusses the different kinds of notes that are written at different stages of the treatment process. From the first notation in the chart that a referral has been received to the closing lines of the discharge summary, occupational therapists (OTs) and OTAs document the many and varied activities of the treatment process. The specific content of the note, the format of the note, and the time lines required vary according to type of setting, accrediting agencies involved, and requirements of third party payers. The contents required for each type of note are described in *Elements of Clinical Documentation* (Revision) (Thomson & Foto, 1995). We will address the requirements for the following kinds of notes.

Initial Evaluation Reports

Before an OTA can begin treatment, the OT must evaluate the patient to determine whether occupational therapy is appropriate for this patient, and if so, what kind of treatment will be most useful. Each setting has its own way of evaluating a patient. A mental health center, for example, may not do the same kind of initial evaluation as a public school or skilled nursing facility. Initial evaluations are usually documented on forms provided by the setting, but may also be done in a SOAP format.

Treatment, Contact, or Visit Notes

Each time treatment is provided by an OT or an OTA, notation is made of what occurred during the treatment session. In some settings, each session is documented using a contact note (also called a treatment note or visit note). In other settings, the therapist makes notes to use later in writing progress notes, but no formalized visit note is required. Many different formats are used for writing contact notes, but in this manual the SOAP format will be taught.

Progress Notes

At the end of a specified period of time, a progress note is written explaining how the patient is responding to treatment and detailing any changes to be made in the treatment plan. Some settings, such as mental health centers, require weekly progress notes. Others, such as residential facilities, require monthly notes. Other settings may use different time periods for reporting. Progress notes may also be written in different formats, but will be taught in a SOAP format in this manual.

Reevaluation Notes

The reevaluation that is part of the occupational therapy treatment process may be documented in a formal reevaluation report in some settings. For example, in a managed care setting, a patient may need to be reevaluated in order to be recertified for treatment after the number of visits initially allocated are completed. This type of note is also the responsibility of the OT, but the experienced OTA may contribute to the reevaluation process (AOTA, 1998).

Discharge Notes

At the end of treatment, a discharge note is written detailing the course of treatment, the accomplishment (or not) of goals, the status at the time of discharge, any home program that may have been recommended, and any other recommendations or referrals. While the OT is responsible for discontinuation of services, an OTA may contribute to the process of discharge under the supervision of the OT (AOTA, 1998). Some settings provide a specific form for the discharge note and other facilities may use the same form that was used for the evaluation. Others use a different format. For purposes of this manual, a SOAP format will be used.

Chapter Nine: Documentation in Different Practice Settings discusses the special requirements of different kinds of practice settings (mental health, long-term care, school-based practice, and critical care pathways), and *Chapter Ten: Making Good Notes Even Better* is a review of what you have learned. Notes from a variety of treatment settings are provided at the end of the manual in *Chapter Eleven: Examples of Different Kinds of Notes*, in addition to the examples scattered throughout the book. The *Appendix: Suggestions for Completing the Worksheets* provides "answers" for the worksheets. However, since there are many "right" ways to answer, these must be viewed as suggestions rather than the only correct answers.

Skilled Occupational Therapy

Throughout this manual, occupational therapy service is described as *skilled occupational therapy*. This term was coined in Medicare regulations, which define the difference between skilled and nonskilled services. Since Medicare Part B requirements are being followed in this manual to insure that your services will not be denied payment, it is important to know that Medicare reimburses those interventions that are identified as skilled and does not reimburse those considered nonskilled. Skilled services are those that require decision-making and highly complex competencies and that have a well-defined knowledge base of human functioning and occupational performance. Nonskilled services are defined as those that are routine or maintenance therapy, both of which could be carried out by nonprofessional personnel or caregivers. The use of "skilled" in this manual emphasizes the necessity of documenting your occupational therapy interventions clearly as those activities requiring the services of a qualified OT or OTA (Lopes, 1998).

Roles of the Occupational Therapist and Occupational Therapy Assistant

The OT and the OTA have different roles and responsibilities in documenting the occupational therapy treatment process. The AOTA provides guidelines in the *Standards of Practice for Occupational Therapy* (AOTA, 1998) and *Occupational Therapy Roles* (AOTA Intercommission Council, 1993) for the responsibilities of different occupational therapy personnel. These guidelines are considered "best practice" but they may differ from state and federal laws that delineate mandatory documentation requirements. Sometimes reimbursement organizations specify who would be an approved documenter for reimbursement purposes. You, as an OTA, are accountable for adhering to the mandatory policies and procedures adopted by state and federal regulatory agencies, but you will find the standards established by AOTA useful in interpreting and following regulations.

The information in this book is intended to provide the OTA with instruction and practice in writing SOAP notes. Specific guidelines for the particular roles of the OT and OTA in documentation of services are dependent upon the specific facility in which the OTA is working. Individual facilities must follow guidelines established by the accrediting agency that governs that facility, for example:

- Joint Commission on Accreditation of Healthcare Organizations (JCAHO)
- Commission on the Accreditation of Rehabilitation Facilities (CARF)
- Comprehensive Outpatient Rehabilitation Facility (CORF)
- Federal and state agencies
- Individual state laws (Backhaus & Sladyk, 2001, p.404; Perinchief, 1998)

In addition, documentation of occupational therapy services must meet with the approval of the third party payers such as Medicare, Medicaid, and/or insurance companies if there is to be reimbursement of those services. All OTAs must have a clear understanding and working knowledge of the requirements that pertain to them in their own particular setting and time. The information that follows can be used as a foundation upon which individual requirements can be built.

According to the *Standards of Practice for Occupational Therapy*, "A certified occupational therapy assistant seeks and follows supervision from a registered OT in the delivery of occupational therapy services" (AOTA, 1998, p. 867). These "occupational therapy services" provided by the OTA will, of course, include documentation of the treatment provided. The level of supervision required is determined by the supervising OT and is based on the skills and demonstrated competency of the OTA, as well as the demands of the job, requirements of the setting, and needs of those receiving treatment (Thomson & Foto, 1995). In general, an entry-level OTA would require close supervision, while the advanced-level OTA who has developed higher skill levels through experience and professional development would require general supervision (AOTA Intercommission Council, 1993). Close supervision would involve direct, daily contact at the work site, while general supervision requires direct contact at least once per month along with other supervision methods (Thomson & Foto, 1995).

Pertaining specifically to documentation, the OT is responsible for performing and documenting the initial evaluation. This evaluation is composed of three parts: identification and background information on the patient, assessment results, and an intervention or treatment plan (AOTA Intercommission Council, 1993). Under the supervision of an OT, the OTA may assist with collecting data for the evaluation or, once competency in the skill has been demonstrated, an OTA at an intermediate or advanced level may administer standardized tests and provide that data to the OT to be considered in the assessment and treatment plan (AOTA, 2000). The role of the experienced OTA is determined by the supervising OT, based on the skills and experience of the OTA, as well as the state licensure regulations (Hirama, 1996).

Contact, Treatment, Visit, and Progress notes are routinely written by OTAs to document the treatments they have provided to individuals receiving skilled occupational therapy. Reevaluation reports involve gathering and assessing current data to determine whether a patient's occupational therapy treatments will continue, be revised, or be discontinued. An OTA may assist in this process by contributing to the reassessment or by performing tasks as requested by the OT (Backhaus & Sladyk, 2001). Once it has been decided that a patient has achieved the goals that have been established (or if those goals cannot be met by the patient) a discharge plan is formulated and a discharge note is written. Again, the OTA may contribute to this process under the supervision of the OT, if not limited or prohibited by mandatory state laws (Hirama, 1996; Fowler, 2001).

In performing the duties of documentation it is crucial the OTA is informed regarding his/her roles and responsibilities. The *Occupational Therapy Code of Ethics*, Principle 5, states that occupational therapy personnel shall,

> *"familiarize themselves with and seek to understand and abide by applicable Association policies; local, state, and federal laws; and institutional rules... and ... remain abreast of revisions in those laws and Association policies that apply to the profession of occupational therapy..."* (AOTA, 2000, p. 615).

Regulations and requirements for documentation by OTA personnel may differ according to the federal and state rules, insurance or Medicare guidelines, and specific facility policies and procedures where they work. Practicing OTAs, whether new graduates or experienced professionals, must accept the ultimate responsibility of keeping their information current in regard to the rules and regulations that will determine their own role in providing appropriate occupational therapy treatments as well as documentation.

Uniform Terminology

Before we discuss documenting the treatment process, we need to differentiate skilled occupational therapy from other disciplines in the health professions. As OTAs, we treat people who have problems in areas of occupational performance. This is important to note, because this is what we will document. The practice of occupational therapy can be divided into performance areas (activities of daily living, work, and leisure) and performance components (the underlying sensory, motor, cognitive, and psychological factors necessary to be independent or successful in the performance areas). In documenting occupational therapy services, the focus on performance areas is critical for showing the necessity for skilled occupational therapy and preventing any question of duplication of services. Skilled occupational therapy may be required to treat functional losses in the following areas.

Activities of Daily Living

There are several levels of activities of daily living, and all of these fall within the scope of skilled occupational therapy. Basic activities of daily living (ADL) are tasks that are necessary for self-care and personal independence, such as bathing, grooming, hygiene, dressing, eating, toileting, communication, and functional mobility. Instrumental activities of daily living (IADL) require more complex problem-solving and social skills and include such tasks as money management, cleaning, laundry, child care, driving, shopping, and meal preparation. Therapists who work with persons with brain injury also talk about executive functions, which are lost in frontal lobe damage. The executive functions include such activities as planning, goal setting, and organizational tasks. In documenting services, it is necessary to demonstrate why a skilled occupational therapy practitioner is needed to perform the task, rather than a family member, aide, or physical therapist (Pedretti, 1996).

In a mental health setting, you would want to consider not just the physical ability to care for self and to interact with the community, but also the emotional components that might be limiting performance. Rather than being limited by a physical factor, a patient with mental illness might be limited by motivation or by the absence of adequate social skills. In a school setting, the ADL tasks of the child are those that allow him to be successful in school, such as the ability to sit still in a chair, hold a pencil, or form letters on a piece of paper.

Work

For younger people, the ability to return to work may be the primary focus of skilled occupational therapy treatment rather than the ability to care for oneself. While Medicare is interested in a person more than 65 years of age being able to perform self-care tasks, workers' compensation is interested in a person less than 65 years being able to return to work. It is important to consider your payment source as well as your patient's interests and priorities as you consider the treatment goals and interventions you plan to use.

Leisure

Those activities that are neither work nor self-care often fall into the category of leisure. Particularly for older people, leisure is a very important part of occupational performance, and yet the limitations of some payment sources may make it a difficult area to document. Often leisure activities are treated by working on the performance components needed for doing the task, rather than approaching the task directly.

Performance Components

Performance components that limit occupational performance also fall within the scope of skilled occupational therapy, as long as there is documentation that a change in the performance component will result in a change in some area of occupational performance. Functional limitations might include such areas as lack of sensory awareness, impaired strength or range of motion, incoordination, abnormal muscle tone, impaired body schema, perceptual deficits, impaired balance or mobility, delusions, disturbances of mood and thought, and environmental barriers. In documenting a treatment session devoted to improving one of these underlying factors, it is critical to tie it to the function that is expected to improve because of the treatment. It is also critical to document in some way that the skill of an OTA was needed to accomplish the task.

Safety Concerns

The ability to perform a task must include the ability to do it safely. Safety concerns such as a high probability of falling, lack of environmental awareness, severe pain (either physical or emotional), the lack of skin sensation, abnormally aggressive or destructive behaviors, or suicide risk all fall within the scope of skilled occupational therapy. Third party payers, such as Medicare, usually see safety as a cost-effective service because it prevents costly further injury.

Prevention of Secondary Complications

Treatment focused on prevention is within the scope of skilled occupational therapy if it can be shown that the patient has a high risk of developing complications. These might include prevention of progressive joint contractures, fracture non-union, and skin breakdown, as well as instruction in joint protection and energy conservation.

Conclusion

In the following pages you will be introduced to the medical record and will learn how to document occupational therapy treatments in the form of SOAP notes. You will find detailed explanations and many opportunities to practice your own writing skills. When you have completed this book and its worksheets you will be prepared to write accurate and concise SOAP notes that will provide the necessary documentation of the occupational therapy treatments you provide as an OTA.

Chapter Two

The Medical Record

Definition and Purpose

The medical record is "a compilation of pertinent facts of a patient's life and health history, including past and present illness(es) and treatment(s), written by the health professionals contributing to that patient's care" (Huffman & Cofer, 1994, p. 28). Like so many other aspects of health care, the medical record is undergoing vast changes as we move further into the information age. The purpose of the record is documentation of the patient's illness and treatment, particularly the current episode. Although the medical record is the physical property of the facility that compiles it, the information contained in the record is actually the property of the patient, and that information must be made available to the patient or to his legal representative upon appropriate request (Huffman & Cofer, 1994).

History

Health care can be traced back approximately 7,000 years to early medicine men who were thought to be able to communicate with the spirit world. Written records can be found as early as 2700 BC in Egypt (Abdelhak, Grostick, Haniken, & Jacobs, 1996). After one of the first hospitals in America was incorporated in Pennsylvania in 1792, its secretary, Benjamin Franklin, began to keep records of patients' names, addresses, disorders, and dates of admission and discharge. These early records were often kept in ledgers, and were brief and handwritten. As medicine advanced, so did the complexity and detail of the medical record. A profession (now called health information management) was created to oversee the record. Most hospitals today are moving toward a computerized record, with a vision that someday paper will no longer be necessary.

The Problem-Oriented Medical Record

In the 1960s a physician named Lawrence Weed decided to reorganize the way medical records were kept (Huffman & Cofer, 1994). He saw the medical record as being arranged for the convenience of the staff, rather than ordered for the highest good of the patient. He developed what he called the Problem-Oriented Medical Record (POMR), which was designed to be a patient-centered method of recording. He wanted to see the record organized into four sections:

1. A database, containing the history and physical, evaluations by all disciplines, lab results, etc.
2. A list of the patient's problems.
3. An interdisciplinary treatment plan, developed by all the staff working with the patient.
4. Progress notes written in chronological order, regardless of discipline.

By organizing the chart in this manner, all information on any of the presenting problems is in one area, easy to find. You don't have to search the chart to see what each discipline has to say about that area of concern. The progress notes are also consolidated rather than being organized by discipline, so that all the information regarding what has happened for/to the patient on that day is in one place. In this way, it is easy for any of the medical staff to read progress notes for the last 24 hours and know everything that is current without having to search several sections of the chart for the necessary information.

As a part of the more patient-centered approach to documentation, Weed recommended that the progress note be organized into four sections including the patient's own perception of the situation, which had heretofore been considered irrelevant. These four sections included:

- **S (Subjective):** the patient's perception of the treatment being received, the progress, limitations, needs, and problems. Normally the subjective section of the note is brief. In an initial evaluation note, however, the "S" might be longer, since it will contain the information the OT obtained in her interview.

- **O (Objective):** the health professional's observations of the treatment being provided. This section will contain all of the measurable, quantifiable, and observable data that was collected from your treatment sessions with the patient. In the initial assessment, the "S" and "O" sections make up the database from which the OT will develop a problem list and treatment plan. Some facilities have combined the first two sections into a composite category called data, and have adapted Weed's SOAP notes into DAP notes. For purposes of this manual, we will continue to use the two discrete sections.

- **A (Assessment):** the health professional's interpretation of the meaning of the events reported in the objective section. In an initial evaluation, the OT will include information in this section on the patient's functional limitations, along with her expectations of the patient's ability to benefit from therapy (sometimes called rehabilitation potential). In a progress note, the assessment component contains explicit statements regarding the patient's progress or lack of progress in therapy. In a problem-oriented record, each progress note is tied to a problem from the patient's problem list, determined by the OT in the initial evaluation.

- **P (Plan):** what the health professional plans to do next to continue with the goals and objectives in the treatment plan. In an initial evaluation, this section contains the treatment plan along with the anticipated frequency and duration of treatment. In a progress note, this is the section where the therapist sets forth the specific treatment, informing the reader what is planned next to help the patient achieve the stated goals.

For almost 30 years, Weed's system was popular in hospitals and rehabilitation centers. Gradually, however, facilities have returned to a more source-oriented medical record, containing sections for each discipline. Even so, the SOAP format of progress notes has remained popular in facilities that no longer use the POMR.

Remember that SOAP is just a format—an outline for organizing information. Any note can be written in this format, although some notes lend themselves to it better than others. For example, you could write a treatment note or discharge summary in a SOAP format, as well as a progress note. You may find that some OTs use this format to write their initial evaluation. However, this format may increase the length of these reports since they also contain a history, summary of functional problems, short- and long-term goals, prior level of functioning, and the beginning treatment plan. For this reason, most practice settings would not use a SOAP format for the initial evaluation report, even if that facility used SOAP for its treatment and progress notes.

The SOAP format is an alternative to narrative notes, which tend to be disorganized and subjective. It forces the writer to look at all four aspects of the treatment session, and to present the information contained in the note in an orderly fashion. A more detailed discussion of each section of the note follows in Chapters Three through Six.

Users and Uses of the Medical Record

The medical record is a communication tool, and has many uses and many different users. It is important to consider all your different audiences when you make an entry in the patient's record.

Patient Care Management

The record is one of the ways the treatment team communicates with each other about the day-to-day aspects of a patient's care. Other therapists in your own department or members of the treatment team will read your notes in order to coordinate care. The OT will communicate the results of the initial evaluation, then your note will provide a report on the patient's progress toward the goals of that initial assessment as well as your plan for continuing care, all of which are important to other members of the treatment team. In a situation where occupational therapy is provided 7 days per week, one OT or OTA may not be providing all of the patient's care and may depend upon the treatment notes to find out what treatment was provided in her absence.

Reimbursement

The medical record is the source document for what services were provided, and for what services may be billed. It is used in billing to substantiate reimbursement claims. For example, if there were a question about the duration and frequency provided, the record would be the source document used to answer that question.

The Legal System

The medical record is a legal document that substantiates what occurred during a patient's illness/treatment. If you have to appear in court to testify, you will be very glad that your documentation is clear and thorough. Sometimes court cases occur years after the event or treatment that is being contested. You may not even remember the event or the patient. What you have written in the medical record will provide you with the information you need in order to testify.

Quality Improvement

Most facilities have a quality improvement (QI) committee whose duty it is to oversee the adequacy and appropriateness of the care that is being provided. This committee is in charge of finding and solving problems in patient care. The medical record is one of the primary sources of information used in the QI process.

Research

The record is also used to provide data for medical research. Some research uses individual data specific to that patient while other research uses aggregate data where no patient name is attached to the data. In either case, the source document is often the medical record.

Accreditation

Accrediting agencies such as the Joint Commission for the Accreditation of Health Care Organizations (JCAHO) and the Commission on Accreditation of Rehabilitation Facilities (CARF) review your notes to ascertain whether the extent and quality of services provided by your facility and/or your department meet the standards of care set by the accrediting agency. If your facility is found to not be in compliance, accreditation may be withdrawn. For example, the Centers for Medicare & Medicaid Services (formerly known as the Health Care Finance Administration or HCFA) accredits facilities that bill for Medicare. If the facility does not meet these standards, all claims that were made by that facility for Medicare services could be denied. The medical record is one of the primary sources of information used during an accreditation visit.

Education

The record may be used as a teaching tool. A student uses the medical record to gain information about patients, as well as about quality and appropriate occupational therapy treatment.

Public Health

The record is also used to identify and to document the incidence of certain diseases, such as tuberculosis or HIV.

Utilization Management

In a hospital setting, the utilization review committee is charged with determining how services in the facility are being utilized. For example, the committee may want to know what kinds of patients are being seen and what kind of care is being provided, and whether these are appropriate to the mission of the facility.

Business Development

Management teams use the information contained in the record to plan and market the services provided by the facility. For example, the director may want to know whether or not there are enough cases of eating disorders being admitted to open a special eating disorders unit.

The Patient

Another significant user is the patient himself. When you are writing in the medical record, always remember that the patient owns the information in his own record and may choose to exercise his right to read what you have written.

Writing in the Record

Since the medical record is not only a communication tool during the patient's hospital stay, but also the source document for financial, legal, and clinical accountability, the record should show the following:

- What services you provided and when.
- What happened and what was said.
- How the client responded to the service provided.
- Why your skill as an OTA was needed rather than the services of an aide or family member.

Before you write anything in the medical record, make these assumptions:

- Someone else will have to read and understand what I write because I may be out sick or out of town the next time this patient needs to be treated.
- The entry I am about to make will be the one scrutinized by a review team from the Centers for Medicare and Medicaid Administration (formerly HCFA) or a Blue Cross representative. If I were a funding source, would I want to pay for the services I am about to record?
- My patient will exercise his right to read this record.

It is critical to know your payment sources when documenting. Some payers are looking for quite different outcomes than others. With a Medicare patient, you will discuss ADLs and write goals for self-care activities. With a workers' compensation case, you will write goals that are oriented to return to work. With home care, you may need to document that your patient is unable to leave home to receive services or that education on safety issues was provided to the caregiver. With a child, you will need to focus on developmental needs or educationally related services identified in the Individualized Education Plan (IEP).

Also remember these facts when planning to write in a patient's record:

- Accuracy is your best protection against problems. You cannot be accurate if you wait too long to record what happened.
- A note in the patient's chart is going to be a reflection of your professional identity and abilities, as well as a reflection of your department and occupational therapy as a profession.
- No activity or contact is ever considered a service that has been provided until a clinical entry is in the record. In terms of fiscal and legal accountability, "If it isn't written, it didn't happen."

Helpful hints on writing notes:

- Be as concise as possible without leaving out pertinent data.
- Avoid generalities.
- Report behavior and avoid judgments except in the assessment portion of your data.
- Be sparse with technical jargon that may be unfamiliar to the reader.

The Mechanics of Documentation

There are a few rules that must be followed when writing in the medical record:

Use Good Grammar

Many of the examples of SOAP notes provided in this book contain incomplete sentences or sentence fragments. In some health care settings this is acceptable, but other facilities may require the use of complete sentences in all documentation. Be sure you check with your supervisor to determine what writing style is expected in your particular facility. In either case you should always use good grammar and correct spelling.

Always Use Waterproof Black Ink

After a certain period of time medical records are microfilmed, and black ink is the only color that microfilms adequately.

Never Use Correction Fluid

Using whiteout in a medical record is considered illegally altering the record. The medical record is a legal document that must stand as originally written.

Correct Errors

If you make an error in the medical record, draw one line through it, write your correction, and initial the change.

> *Pt. able to dress lower body with ~~verbal cues~~ SB min Ⓐ using a reacher.*

In a problem-oriented medical chart, if you inadvertently write your note in the wrong patient's chart, draw a single line through the entire entry and write "wrong chart" beside it with your signature.

If you need to add something after you have written and signed your note, write an addendum with the current date and time.

Be Sure All Required Data is Present

The *Elements of Clinical Documentation* (Revision) (Thomson & Foto, 1995) and *The Guide to Occupational Therapy Practice* (Moyers, 1999) specify the contents for each type of note you may be writing. This information will be covered in Chapter Eight. Make certain that your note contains all the necessary information, and remember, **it is absolutely critical that you sign and date your note.** In some situations, when required by law or the facility, documentation written by an OTA will need to be co-signed by a registered OT (Thomson & Foto, 1995). The notes we have provided in this book were submitted by students, OTAs, and OTs, who gave their permission to use their notes as examples. We have not ended every note with the therapist's name and date in order to maintain confidentiality.

Be Concise

In today's health care system, busy professionals are often pressed for time and appreciate being able to read what you have written in the shortest time possible. Your own time for documentation will also be limited under today's productivity standards.

Use Appropriate Terminology for the Recipients of Services

When referring to the people who use occupational therapy services, we have traditionally referred to them as patients or clients based on the setting where services were received. However, as practice areas are rapidly changing and expanding, the AOTA has addressed the use of terminology in the official document *Service Delivery in Occupational Therapy* (AOTA, 1995) as follows:

> *Service provision occurs directly with individuals, groups, programs, or organizations. Depending on the setting in which the occupational therapy practitioner works, various terms may be used for individual clients (e.g., patient, consumer, resident, participant, student, teacher, employer, or administrator). Group clients may include families, teams, or others with common needs. (p. 98)*

For the purposes of this manual, names have been fabricated to protect the privacy of those people who receive our services. The terms patient, consumer, client, resident, individual, and veteran, as well as first names have been used. In a note that says "Mr. P. was seen in his home..." please understand that he is being called "Mr. P." for purposes of confidentiality. In your note, you would use his whole name.

Use Approved Abbreviations

Use only the abbreviations that are approved by your facility. While it saves time to use symbols and abbreviations, remember that your notes may be read by someone with a high school education who knows little about occupational therapy and who will determine whether or not to pay for your services. It is wise to be sure that the person is able to understand what you have written. Your facility will be able to furnish a list of the abbreviations it allows so the abbreviations and symbols you use will be validated if there is a question. Do not make up your own abbreviations, and do not use any abbreviation that is not on your facility's approved list. Remember, it is permitted to use abbreviations, but it is not necessary. You are permitted to write out any word instead of shortening it. In this manual you will find that some notes use more abbreviations and symbols than others. (See Table 2-1 for suggested symbols and abbreviations.)

Table 2-1
Abbreviations and Symbols

A	anterior; assessment
Ⓐ	assistance
ā	before
AAROM	active assistive range of motion
ABI	acquired brain injury
a.c.	before meals
abd	abduction
ACTH	adrenocorticotrophic hormone
add	adduction
ADD	Attention Deficit Disorder
ADHD	Attention Deficit Hyperactivity Disorder
ADL	activity of daily living
ad lib.	as desired
AIDS	acquired immunodeficiency syndrome
AE	above elbow
AK	above knee
AKA	above knee amputation
am, AM	morning
AMA	against medical advice
amb	ambulation
amt	amount
AP	anterior-posterior
AROM	active range of motion
ASA	aspirin
ASAP	as soon as possible
ASHD	arteriosclerotic heart disease
ASIS	anterior superior iliac spine
Ⓑ	bilateral
BE	below elbow
b.i.d.	twice a day
BK	below knee
BKA	below knee amputation
BM	bowel movement
BP	blood pressure
BRP	bathroom privileges
BS	blood sugar
B/S	bedside
BUN	blood urea nitrogen
Bx	biopsy
c̄	with
C	Celsius; centigrade
CA	carcinoma; cancer
C&S	culture and sensitivity
CABG	coronary artery bypass graft
CAD	coronary artery disease
cal	calories
cap	capsule
CAT	computerized axial tomography
CBC	complete blood count
cc	cubic centimeter
CC	chief complaint
CCU	coronary (cardiac) care unit
CGA	contact guard assist
CHF	congestive heart failure
CHI	closed head injury
cm	centimeter
CNS	central nervous system
CO_2	carbon dioxide
c/o	complains of
cont.	continue
cmc, CMC	carpometacarpal
COPD	chronic obstructive pulmonary disease
COTA	certified occupational therapy assistant
CP	cerebral palsy
CPR	cardiopulmonary resuscitation
CSF	cerebrospinal fluid
CT	computed tomography
CTR	carpal tunnel release
cu mm	cubic millimeter
CVA	cerebrovascular accident
CXR	chest x-ray
d	day
Ⓓ	dependent
D&C	dilation and curettage
d/c, DC, D/C	discharge; discontinue
D.C.	doctor of chiropractic medicine
D.D.S.	doctor of dental surgery
DIP	distal interphalangeal joint
DJD	degenerative joint disease
DLS	daily living skills
D.O.	doctor of osteopathic medicine
DM	diabetes mellitus
dr	dram
Dr.	doctor
DTR	deep tendon reflex
DVT	deep vein thrombosis
Dx	diagnosis
ECG	electrocardiogram
ECHO	echocardiogram
EEG	electroencephalogram
EKG	electrocardiogram
EMG	electromyogram
ENT	ear, nose, throat
EOB	edge of bed
ER	emergency room
ETOH	ethyl alcohol
eval.	evaluation
ext.	extension
F	Fahrenheit; Fair (muscle strength grade of 3)
f	female
F.A.C.P.	fellow of the American College of Physicians
F.A.C.S.	fellow of the American College of Surgeons
FBS	fasting blood sugar
FH	family history
flex.	flexion
fl oz	fluid ounce
FROM	functional range of motion
FSH	follicle-stimulating hormone
ft.	foot, feet (the measurement, not the body part)
FUO	fever, unknown origin
FWB	full weight bearing
Fx	fracture
G	Good (muscle strength grade of 4)
GB	gallbladder
GI	gastrointestinal
gm	gram
g, gr	grain
GTT	glucose tolerance test
GYN	gynecology
h	hour
HA, H/A	headache
H&P	history and physical
HBV	hepatitis B virus
HCT, Hct	hematocrit
HEENT	head, eyes, ears, nose, throat
HEP	home exercise program
HGB, Hgb	hemoglobin
HIV	human immunodeficiency virus

Table 2-1 continued
Abbreviations and Symbols

HOB	head of bed
HRT	hormone replacement therapy
HR	heart rate
hr.	hour
hs	at bedtime
Ht	height
HTN	hypertension
Hx	history
Ⓘ	independent
IADL	instrumental activity of daily living
ICU	intensive care unit
IDDM	insulin-dependent diabetes mellitus
IM	intramuscular
IMP	impression
in.	inches
IP	inpatient
IUD	intrauterine device
IV	intravenous
kg	kilogram
KUB	kidney, ureter, bladder
Ⓛ	left; liter
L	left
lb, #	pound
LE	lower extremity
LLQ	left lower quadrant
LP	lumbar puncture
LTG	long-term goal
LUQ	left upper quadrant
m	murmur; meter; male
max	maximum
Meds.	medications
MFT	muscle function test
MD	muscular dystrophy; medical doctor
mg	milligram
MI	myocardial infarction
ml	milliliter
min	minutes; minimum
mm	millimeter
mo.	month
mod	moderate
MP, MCP	metacarpophalangeal
MRI	magnetic resonance imaging
MS	multiple sclerosis; musculoskeletal
MSH	melanocyte-stimulating hormone
MVP	mitral valve prolapse
N	Normal (muscle strength grade of 5)
NDT	neurodevelopmental treatment
neg.	negative
NG	nasogastric
NKA	no known allergy
NKDA	no known drug allergy
noc.	night
NPO	nothing by mouth
NSR	normal sinus rhythm
NWB	non-weightbearing
O	objective; oriented
O_2	oxygen
Ox4	oriented to time, place, person, situation
OB	obstetrics
OBS	organic brain syndrome
OH	occupational history
OP	outpatient
OR	operating room
ORIF	open reduction, internal fixation
OT	occupational therapist; occupational therapy
OTA	occupational therapy assistant
OTR	occupational therapist, registered
oz	ounce
p̄	after
P	plan; posterior; pulse; Poor (muscle strength grade of 2)
PA	posterior anterior; physician's assistant
PAP	Papanicolaou test (smear)
PDD	Pervasive Developmental Disorder
PE	physical examination
per	by
PET	positron emission tomography
PFT	pulmonary function testing
Ph.D.	doctor of philosophy
PID	pelvic inflammatory disease
PIH	pregnancy induced hypertension
PIP	proximal interphalangeal
p.m., PM	afternoon
PMH	past medical history
PNF	proprioceptive neuromuscular facilitation
PNI	peripheral nerve injury
PNS	peripheral nervous system
p.o.	by mouth
POMR	problem-oriented medical record
pos.	positive
poss	possible
post op	post operation
pre op	pre operation
p.r.n.	as needed
pro	pronation
PROM	passive range of motion
pt.	patient
PT	physical therapist, physical therapy
PTA	physical therapist assistant; prior to admission
PTCA	percutaneous transluminal coronary angioplasty
PTH	parathyroid hormone
PWB	partial weight bearing
Px	physical examination
q	every
qd	every day
qh	every hour
q2h	every two hours
q.i.d.	four times a day
qn	every night
q.o.d.	every other day
qt.	quart
R	right; respiration
Ⓡ	right
RA	rheumatoid arthritis
RBC	red blood cell count
R.D.	registered dietician
re:	regarding
rehab	rehabilitation
resp	respiratory; respiration
RLQ	right lower quadrant
R/O	rule out
ROM	range of motion
ROS	review of symptoms
RROM	resistive range of motion

Table 2-1 continued
Abbreviations and Symbols

R.T.	respiratory therapist; recreation therapist
RTC	return to clinic
RTO	return to office
RUQ	right upper quadrant
RSD	reflex sympathetic dystrophy
Rx	recipe; Latin *take thou prescription*
s̄	without
S	subjective
SBA	stand by assistance
SH	social history
Sig:	instruction to patient
SLE	systemic lupus erythematosus
SOC	start of care
SOAP	subjective objective assessment plan
SOB	shortness of breath
SNF	skilled nursing facility
SpGr	specific gravity
S/P	status post
sq	subcutaneous
SR	systems review
STAT	immediately
STD	sexually transmitted disease
STG	short-term goal
suppos	suppository
sup	supination
Sx	symptom
T	temperature; Trace (muscle strength grade of 1)
T&A	tonsillectomy and adenoidectomy
tab	tablet
TAB	therapeutic abortion
TB	tuberculosis
TBI	traumatic brain injury
tbsp.	tablespoon
TDWB	touch-down weightbearing
TEDS	thromboembolic disease stockings
TENS, TNS	transcutaneous electrical nerve stimulator
THR	total hip replacement
TIA	transient ischemic attack
t.i.d.	three times a day
TKR	total knee replacement
TM(J)	temporomandibular (joint)
TNR	tonic neck reflex (also ATNR; STNR)
t.o.	telephone order
TPR	temperature, pulse, and respiration
TRS	therapeutic recreation specialist
tsp.	teaspoon
TSH	thyroid-stimulating hormone
tx	treatment; traction
TTWB	toe-touch weight bearing
UA	urinalysis
UE	upper extremity
UMN	upper motor neuron
URI	upper respiratory infection
US	ultrasound
UTI	urinary tract infection
UV	ultraviolet
VC	vital capacity
VD	venereal disease
v.o.	verbal orders
vol.	volume
VS	vital signs
WBAT	weight bearing as tolerated
WBC	white blood cell; white blood count
w/c	wheelchair
WDWN	well developed, well nourished
wk	week
WFL	within functional limits
WNL	within normal limits
wt	weight
w/w	wheeled walker
x2	assistance (assistance of 2 persons given; also written "assistance of 2") Example: "transferred to toilet c̄ max Ⓐ x2"
y.o.	year old
yd.	yard
yr	year
♂	male
♀	female
↓	down; downward; decrease
↑	up; upward; increase
~	approximately
@	at
Δ	change
>	greater than
<	less than
=	equals
+	plus; positive (also abbreviated pos.)
-	minus; negative (also abbreviated neg.)
#	number (#1); pounds
/	per
%	percent
+, &, et.	and
°	degree
✓	flexion
/	extension
⇆, ↔	to and from
→	to; progressing forward; approaching
1°	primary
2°	secondary; secondary to

Worksheet 2-1

Using Abbreviations

Translate each sentence written with abbreviations into full English phrases or sentences using Table 2-1.

Pt. c/o pain in Ⓡ MCP joint $\bar{p}$ ~15 min PROM.

Pt. w/c → mat $\bar{c}$ sliding board max Ⓐ x2.

Pt. Ox4.

Pt. able to don pants SBA $\bar{c}$ verbal cues to thread Ⓛ LE.

1° dx. THR 2° dx. COPD & CHF.

Shorten these notes using only the standard abbreviations in this chapter.

Patient has thirty degrees of passive range of motion in the left distal interphalangeal joint, which is within functional limits.

Patient is able to put on her socks with standby assistance, but requires moderate assistance with putting on and taking off left shoe.

The patient requires contact guard assistance for balance during her morning dressing, which she performs while sitting on the edge of her bed.

Worksheet 2-2

Additional Practice

Shorten these notes using the standard abbreviations provided in Table 2-1.

The patient was seen bedside for training in activities of daily living. She was able to perform bed mobility exercises with moderate assistance, but needed maximum assistance to put on her Depends (Kimberly-Clarke Corp., Dallas, TX). She was able to go from a supine position to a sitting position with minimum assistance and from a sitting position to a standing position with moderate assistance.

The resident came to the occupational therapy clinic via wheelchair escort. The resident was observed to lean to his left. The resident needed verbal cues and minimum assistance in positioning his body in the wheelchair to maintain midline orientation and symmetrical posture. The resident transferred from his wheelchair to the toilet with moderate assistance of one person using a standing pivot transfer. He needed verbal cues and visual feedback from a mirror to maintain upright posture.

The veteran has been treated three out of five times in the past week. Two treatments were missed due to urinary tract infection. The veteran's short-term memory was three out of three for immediate recall, one out of three after one minute, and zero out of three with verbal cues after five minutes. The left upper extremity shoulder flexion was a grade of four, shoulder extension was a grade of four, elbow flexion was a grade of four, elbow extension was a grade of four, wrist extension was a grade of three minus, wrist flexion was a grade of three minus, and grip strength was at eight pounds. The right upper extremity muscle grades are within normal limits.

The patient is a sixty-three year old female who had coronary artery bypass graft surgery. Her past medical history includes diabetes mellitus type 2, hypertension, coronary artery disease, and degenerative joint disease. Her discharge date from the skilled nursing home was April 1, 2001.

Chapter Three

Writing the "S"—Subjective

The first section of the SOAP note contains **SUBJECTIVE** information obtained from the patient, giving his perspective on his condition or treatment. Subjective data is information that cannot be verified or measured during your treatment session. In this section the therapist records the patient's report of limitations, concerns, and problems. This is where you document what the patient said that was relevant to treatment, such as significant complaints of pain, fatigue, or expressions of feelings, attitudes, concerns, goals, and plans. When direct quotes are used in the subjective section of the SOAP note, it is understood that the statement comes from the individual receiving the therapy, unless otherwise stated.

The information obtained from the patient will be of greater significance and relevance to the rest of your note if it is specific rather than general in nature. For instance, if the patient tells you, "My shoulder hurts," you may question him further, asking him "where does it hurt?" or "when does it hurt?", so your note can communicate more detailed information on his condition, writing "Patient states his Ⓡ shoulder hurts when he tries to put his shirt on." You may use a quote or summarize what the patient said.

Examples of "S" statements:

- Pt. communicated using her message board that she wanted to be able to take care of herself.
- "I don't need therapy."
- Resident reports pain in Ⓡ shoulder when reaching up to comb hair.
- Patient asked for help when it was needed during dressing.
- "I can't wash the dishes or zip my coat."
- Veteran reports that his fingers "look kind of dead."
- Pt. reported he needed to go to meet someone and get to work when the session began. When asked questions such as "can you hear me?" he often responded, "I need to go."
- Resident reports he feels "pretty good" now and his goal is to "get back as natural" as he can.
- Pt. reports that his doctor has ordered some home care for "a few days to work on transfers."
- During the initial occupational therapy session, client reported, "I keep blowing up at home, and yelling at everyone, and I don't know what to do about it."
- Client reported that her shoulders feel better after taping. "My short-term goal is to return to work, and my long-term goal is to be able to write."
- Pt. described her previous medical history, including the fall that fractured her Ⓡ ankle. She reports living with her daughter and having an attendant stay with her when her daughter is at work. Pt. reports having a hospital bed as well as a trapeze, walker, and 3-in-1 commode. She reports having four steps leading into her home, with handrails on both sides.
- Resident reports being able to bathe and dress self Ⓘ, but does not open dresser drawers and closet doors due to a fall from opening a dresser drawer which resulted in a hip fracture. She was able to tell the correct day and month when asked.
- Patient commented that she used her Ⓛ hand to hold a cup but now is unable to do so. Pt. also inquired about finding a student to assist her at home upon discharge. Patient also complained of soreness in Ⓛ shoulder and stated that she has experienced several episodes of bladder incontinence when trying to make it to the bathroom.
- Martha called the emergency line last night to report a burning sensation in her "gut" which made her afraid she was going to die. Today she reports that she has been worrying about dying and has not showered since the day before yesterday.

- Consumer contributed to ~98% of the group discussion, reporting that the hardest feelings for her to deal with are worry and fear about her physical problems, which might go undetected. She reports being unable to function at home (cannot cook, keep house, or do laundry) when she is sick with depression, but wants to do these things again. Consumer reports that exercise, prayer, and volunteer work are her primary coping strategies, and that she would like to learn more about relaxation techniques.

Sometimes the patient is not able to speak or does not make any relevant comments. In such cases, include that information in the "S" section.

For example:

- Patient unable to communicate due to aphasia.
- Patient did not speak without cuing.
- Resident does not clearly verbalize during treatment, but smiles and nods appropriately when asked questions.

Occasionally you will include information that the nursing staff or family provided about the patient if this is pertinent to the note or patient's progress. However, the "S" section is usually reserved for the patient's view.

Common Errors

Not Using Communication Time With the Patient Effectively

The most common error that new therapists make in gathering subjective information is in failing to make good use of communication time with the patient during treatment sessions. Instead of using the time in therapy to talk socially, a good therapist will use the time to listen effectively and ask questions that will provide pertinent information about the patient's attitudes and concerns that can be used to ensure appropriate documentation as well as effective treatment. Instead of talking to your patient about the weather or Monday Night Football, why not ask him how he thinks he is doing in therapy or what his feelings are related to his upcoming discharge to home? As therapists gain experience, they begin to use the treatment session to provide relevant data regarding such things as functional status, prior level of functioning, motivation, priorities, and family support.

Effective communication and interviewing during treatment sessions can seem just like a conversation on the surface. However, as a skilled therapist you are directing the conversation to topics that are meaningful to patient care rather than allowing it to remain superficial. Use this opportunity to update and gather data that is vital to providing the very best occupational therapy possible. In having a conversation with your patient, guide the discussion to your patient's history, problems, needs, strengths, support systems, living situation, and goals for treatment. Without knowing these things from your patient's point of view, you will have difficulty planning effective treatment. When a therapist does not listen effectively during treatment, the "S" may read:

- Patient talked about grandchildren visiting. - OR - Pt. said "ouch" when elbow was ranged beyond 45°.

While these statements are within the scope of the "S," they are not particularly helpful pieces of information to spend time and space reporting.

Not Writing Concise, Coherent Statements

The second most common error made by new therapists in writing the subjective section of the note is that of simply listing any remarks the patient makes about his condition.

For example, during one treatment session the patient may make the following statements:

- "I can't feel anything with my hands."
- "I'm wobbly as all get out today."
- Pt. expressed dizziness after bending down to touch the floor while in a seated position. Pt. acknowledged improvement in his sitting balance in comparison to the previous week.

While these statements can provide objective, relevant data regarding the patient's stability, balance, and safety, they have no coherence when they are strung together as a list of separate remarks made by the patient during his treatment. It is more effective to summarize the patient's remarks in a concise and coherent manner, instead of listing each of these statements separately in the "S" section of the note.

For example:

- Pt. expressed lack of sensation in both hands and dizziness in sitting position with dynamic movement (a "wobbly" sensation). He also acknowledged improvement in sitting balance since last week.

Worksheet 3-1

Writing Concise, Coherent Statements

During a treatment session your patient makes the following statements.

- "I used that dressing stick and sock aid like you showed me to get dressed without bending down this morning."
- "My hip doesn't hurt when I stand up or sit down, especially with that new toilet seat you got for me."
- "It's getting easier for me to get dressed now."
- "My daughter said they delivered all that bathroom equipment to her house yesterday."

Using these statements, write your own concise and organized version for the "S" portion of the SOAP note.

Worksheet 3-2

Choosing a Subjective Statement

An OTA student wrote the following observation after treating a patient:

Pt. seen in rehab clinic for UE activities to ↑ AROM in Ⓡ shoulder, activity tolerance, UE strength, and dynamic standing balance, in order to ↑ independence in ADL tasks.

ADL: Pt. seen in room for instruction in safety techniques and adaptive equipment use in toileting. Pt. needs bilateral grab bars in bathroom to sit ↔ stand safely. Pt. attempted to stand while pulling on walker and one grab bar. Pt. was instructed on safety issues and the use of bilateral grab bars.

Performance Components: Pt. sit ↔ stand CGA for balance. Pt. worked on activity tolerance, dynamic standing balance, and ↑ AROM in Ⓡ shoulder by moving canned goods from counter to cupboard for 5 minutes before needing a 2-minute sitting rest. After resting, participated in activities to ↑ dynamic standing balance by pouring liquid from a pitcher while standing CGA for balance. After a 1-minute rest, pt. continued activities to ↑ dynamic standing balance and safety in ADL activities by pushing wheeled walker while picking up objects from floor c̄ a reacher. AROM in right shoulder abduction <90°. PROM Ⓡ shoulder abduction WNL.

The treatment session included all of the following. Which would be best to use as the subjective section of the SOAP note?

- Patient was cooperative and engaged in social conversation throughout the treatment session.
- Patient remarked that her grandson will be coming to visit later in the week, and that she will be very glad to see him.
- Patient reports that she feels "pretty good" today.
- Patient says she is unable to move Ⓡ UE, although she does not know why it will not move. She reports, "It really doesn't hurt. It's just tight."
- Nursing staff report patient is unsafe to toilet self independently.

Chapter Four

Writing the "O" — Objective

The second section of the note is **OBJECTIVE**—where you will record all measurable, quantifiable, and observable data obtained during the treatment session. You can also include the length of the treatment session here, since many insurance companies will require this information in your note.

In this section you will present a picture of the treatment session you have observed. When you look at things with your professional eyes, you begin to see things differently. Instead of seeing a child playing with a toy, now you begin to note the child's asymmetrical posture, his bilateral hand use, ability to cross midline, and his pinch and grasp patterns. The trick in writing the "O" is in knowing what kind of material to include and what to omit. At first your "O" may tend to be longer than that of an experienced therapist, but with time you will learn to write notes that are both complete and concise.

Organization of the "O"

There are different ways that are acceptable in organizing the information in your observation. You may choose to present the information chronologically, discussing each treatment event in the order it occurred during that treatment session. For example:

O: Pt. seen for 45 minutes in clinic for wheelchair positioning. Foot-guard attached to prevent Ⓛ foot from dropping behind/between footrests. New wedge cushion c̄ dycem inserted on both sides to prevent slipping. Wedge pillow placed on Ⓛ side for lateral support. Folded blanket placed between pt.'s knees. Family (via a phone call) and staff educated on pt.'s positioning changes and goals.

Alternately, you may choose to organize your information into categories.

O: Pt. seen for 1 hour in clinic kitchen for skilled instruction in compensatory techniques for cooking.

Mobility: Pt. maneuvered throughout kitchen in w/c with verbal cues to place w/c in appropriate position for reaching objects in kitchen. Pt. min Ⓐ in stabilizing items while transporting items in lap and maneuvering w/c simultaneously.

UE AROM and strength: WFL for reaching items in drawers, opening oven door, and putting dishes in the sink Ⓘ. UE strength adequate for opening refrigerator door and stirring batter Ⓘ. Pt. requires min Ⓐ in opening Tupperware container.

Hand function and strength: Adequate for unscrewing lids, cracking egg, and opening muffin box Ⓘ. Pt. able to use necessary tools for carrying out task Ⓘ. Pt. able to set oven dial and put muffins in oven Ⓘ.

Activity tolerance: Pt. took 3-minute break after ~20 minutes of activity Ⓘ.

Cognition: Pt. able to respond to verbal instructions and questions with correct response 3/3 times. Pt. said she did not think it would be safe for her to take the muffins out of the oven. Pt. able to problem-solve Ⓘ about repositioning her w/c 75% of tx time.

When categorizing your information, choose the categories that make sense for your note. There is no list of "correct" categories. You may choose to report the treatment session chronologically or divide your information into categories. If the patient has not had deficits in one of these areas, it is not necessary to include that category in the note, unless it is becoming a problem.

You may want to consider including some of the following categories in your observation of physical disability (O'Hara, 1990):

- Specifics of ADL performance: setting of the session, type of clothing, shaver, etc. Include assist levels and set-up needed, any adaptive equipment or technique used, UE or LE. Also include type of cuing and response, family education, positioning, special equipment, and how the various performance components affect function.
- Assist levels: note what part of the activity required your assistance (for example, "min Ⓐ for balance") as well as what part of the activity required verbal cues (for example, "verbal cues to position walker safely").
- The patient's posture and balance: consider whether the patient leans in one direction, has rotated posture, even or uneven weight distribution. Notice position of the head, facial expression, and symmetry.
- The patient's coordination: hand dominance, type of prehension used, ability to grasp and maintain grasp without dropping, gross vs. fine motor ability.
- Swelling or edema: give girth or volumetric measurements if possible, pitting or non-pitting, including levels if pitting.
- Movement patterns observed in affected upper extremity: tone, tremors, synergy pattern, facilitation required, stabilization, body movement.
- Ability to follow instructions: type and amount of instruction required, such as physical, verbal, or visual cuing, ability to follow one, two, or three step directions.
- The patient's cognitive status: initiation of task, verbal responses, approach to the task, ability to stay on task, sequencing, oriented x4 (identifying time, place, person, and situation), requirements for cuing, number of steps successfully completed in task, judgment (recognition of impairments, impulsivity), ability to respond to written or verbal directions.
- Neurological factors: perseveration (motor, speech), sensory losses (specific), motor deficit, praxis, damage to innervation (spasticity, flaccidity, rigidity, synergy), unilateral neglect, bilateral integration, tremors.
- Performance components: ROM (active, passive, assistive) and why limited, strength (grade and extremity), endurance (time, repetition, signs of fatigue, sitting/standing), dexterity (one- or two-handed, grip, grasp and release, object manipulation), speed of task completion, sensation.
- The patient's mobility status: what kind of assistance is needed for the patient to walk or propel his wheelchair (equipment, adapted technique, stand-by, verbal cues).

Observations in Different Practice Settings

In a mental health setting you will be observing psychosocial factors as well as functional ability. For example:

Client attended anger management group for 45 minutes today with verbal prompting by nursing staff and security aides. He displayed his displeasure at being asked to attend the group by using profanity. During the group, client related two instances in which individuals on the unit consistently bothered him, and discussed the way he usually handles this situation. Peer feedback was given on other possible ways he might handle the same situation.

In this setting you may use some of the following categories in your note (Mason, 2001):

- Social Interaction: awareness of others in the group, length of conversations, initiation of conversation, interaction with peers or leader in a group setting.
- Judgment and Problem-Solving: impulsivity, safety awareness, ability to identify and correct errors.
- Behavior: agitation, lethargy, affect, compulsivity, anxiety, demanding behavior.
- Appearance: grooming, choice of appropriate attire.
- Work Skills: promptness, concentration, attention span, ability to follow direction, organization of task, including preparation and clean up.

In a pediatric setting, the child's play or school activities are a part of her activities of daily living.

Mary was seen in her home for 50 minutes to work on Ⓑ tasks to ↑ spontaneous use of Ⓛ hand as a functional assist, as well as sitting balance as prerequisites to Ⓘ in self-care and play skills.

- Bilateral UE Use: Mary required mod Ⓐ to pull shirt over stuffed animal's arm. She spontaneously used Ⓛ hand to pull/stabilize animal while pulling shirt over its arm and shoulder with Ⓡ hand. She initiated snapping shirt, and used Ⓑ UEs to hold shirt, but required max Ⓐ to fasten snaps. Mary used both hands to hold animal during play.
- Sitting balance: Mary requires touch cues stand ↔ sit in walker, and mod physical Ⓐ sit → cross-leg sit. She demonstrated adequate sitting balance to play for 5 minutes, but after 5 minutes needed 2 tactile cues to sit up from forward leaning position.

In the school system, all activities must be related to school functioning.

Student was seen in classroom to work on letter recognition and formation. After proprioceptive input, she was able to identify and match upper and lower case letters with 90% accuracy and min verbal cues to verbalize answers. She required mod verbal cues and demonstration to form lower case letters correctly.

The Specifics of Writing the "O"

Begin With a Statement About the Setting and Purpose of the Activity

Pt. seen for ____ minutes ______________________________ for ______________________________.
(In what setting) (Purpose of the treatment session)

Some third party payers will require documentation of the length of time of the treatment session. You will need to check with your facility to determine whether this needs to be included in your note.

If the session is centered on working on performance components such as strengthening, range of motion, activity tolerance, or dynamic balance, then add a reference to the relevant performance area in the opening sentence:

Patient seen _____________ for _________________, ______________________________________.
(Setting) (Purpose) (For what expected functional gain)

For example:

- "Pt. seen for 45 minutes in occupational therapy clinic to address Ⓛ side neglect and impaired motor planning in self-care activities."
- "Patient seen in dayroom on unit for instruction in anger management techniques needed to maintain relationships and employment."
- "Client seen for 60 minutes in room to provide skilled instruction in energy conservation in IADL activities and for explanation of patient education materials on energy conservation."
- "Joe participated in collage activity for 30 minutes in assertion group in order to explore and share feelings re: hospitalization."
- "Patient seen in outpatient clinic to increase functional movements and prehension patterns of Ⓛ hand in order to prepare for return to work."
- "Child seen for ½ hour in therapy room to ↑ strength and tone needed to improve handwriting."
- "Student seen in sensory integration playroom to address sensory defensiveness in classroom activities."

It is helpful to show the need for your skill as an OTA in the very first sentence of your "O." For example, instead of saying "Pt. seen bedside for ADL training," you might say:

- "Pt. seen bedside for instruction in compensatory dressing techniques."
- "Resident seen for 45 minutes bedside for instruction in use of adaptive equipment to increase safety in ADL tasks."
- "Veteran seen for ½ hour bedside to facilitate attention to Ⓛ side during self-care activities. "

Follow the Opening Sentence of the "O" With a Chronological Rendition of the Session, Such As:

O: Client seen in his home and taken on city bus for community re-integration following discharge from inpatient facility. By simulation, client demonstrated home management skills and ability to care for animals. Client was able to identify which bus to catch to go to grocery store, but needed reassurance that his choice was correct. At the grocery store, client chose lunchmeat and fruit for lunches this week, but needed SBA for payment.

Or a Categorized Summary, Such As:

O: Patient seen in rehab gym for UE activities to ↑ AROM in shoulder, activity tolerance, UE strength, and dynamic standing balance, in order to ↑ Ⓘ in ADL activities.

ADL: Pt. seen for 30 minutes in room for instruction in safety techniques and adaptive equipment use in toileting. Pt. needs bilateral grab bars in bathroom to sit ↔ stand safely. Patient attempted to stand while pulling on walker and one grab bar. Patient was instructed on safety issues and the use of bilateral grab bars.

Performance components: Pt. sit ↔ stand CGA for balance. Pt. worked on activity tolerance, dynamic standing balance and ↑ AROM in right shoulder by moving canned goods from counter to cupboard for 5 minutes before needing a 2-minute sitting rest. After resting, participated in activities to ↑ dynamic standing balance by pouring liquid from a pitcher while standing CGA for balance. After a 1-minute rest, pt. continued activities to ↑ dynamic standing balance and safety in ADL activities by pushing wheeled walker while picking up objects from the floor with a reacher. AROM in right shoulder abduction <90°. PROM right shoulder abduction WNL.

Some notes work better if they are divided into categories. Consider the following observation:

- Child seen for 60 minutes in daycare setting to work on reach/grasp/release and feeding skills. With min Ⓐ for facilitation of movement at elbow, child demonstrated ability to use Ⓛ UE to reach, grasp, and release 5 objects with 1 to 2 verbal cues per object and restriction of Ⓡ UE movement. Child was able to feed self Ⓘ c̄ ~50% spillage, but demonstrated significant limitations in chewing action c̄ ~3 rotary chews & swallowing ~90% of food without chewing. Child required verbal cues throughout session to maintain attention to task. Child wore soft spica thumb splint for entire tx session.

How would you divide this information into categories to make it easier to read? Write your categories in the box below:

Worksheet 4-1

Choosing Categories

In Writing Your "O", Focus on the Patient's Response to the Treatment Provided, Rather Than What You Did.

Rather than saying:	"Patient was reminded about hip precautions."
You might say:	"Attempting to don shoes, pt. required repeated instruction to keep hip in correct alignment."
Rather than saying:	"Patient was asked orientation questions pertaining to the time of day."
You might say:	"When verbally cued to look at watch, patient was unable to correctly identify time."
Rather than saying:	"Patient demonstrated a postural drift backward and to the left several times while sitting on the edge of the mat."
You might say:	"Patient required verbal and tactile cues to correct postural drift backward and to the left 4 times in 5 minutes while sitting edge of mat."

Always Write from the Patient's Point of View, Leaving Yourself Out

Rather than saying:	"The OTA put the patient's shoes on for him."
You might say:	"Pt. Ⓓ in donning shoes."
Rather than saying:	"OTA instructed the client and family in energy conservation techniques."
You might say:	"Client and family instructed in energy conservation techniques and demonstrated understanding by performing correctly."

Make Certain That it is Clear That You Were Not Just a Passive Observer in the Session

Rather than saying:	"Client compensated for shoulder flexion by leaning forward with whole body during prehension activities."
You might say:	"Client required skilled instruction to avoid compensation at the shoulder during prehension activities."
Rather than saying:	"Patient performed Home Exercise Program."
You might say:	"Home Exercise Program was observed for accurate movement patterns and updated to accommodate for progress."

Although You Will Assess the Information You Observed and Make a Professional Judgment About it, Avoid Judging the Patient

Rather than saying:	"Patient was compliant." or "Patient was cooperative."
You might say:	"Patient demonstrated ability to follow 3-step directions and sequence WFL."

Be Professional and Concise in Your Wording

Rather than saying:	"Veteran used a trapeze to sit up."
You might say:	"Supine → sit using trapeze."
Rather than saying:	"Client placed the board to make a sliding board transfer."
You might say:	"Client positioned sliding board for transfer."
Rather than saying:	"Resident flopped down onto bed short of breath, closed her eyes and moaned. Resident laid in bed with min Ⓐ to position herself."
You might say:	"Pt. observed to be fatigued following tx session and required min Ⓐ for positioning in bed."

Focus on Function

Make certain that function is integral to the note. In a treatment session devoted to self-care activities, function is obvious. However, in a session devoted to treating performance components such as strength, range, and endurance or in a session where modalities are used or in a co-treatment session, **function must be addressed** separately in order to justify skilled occupational therapy. For example, although the note below is an observation of a session that was devoted to performance components, it contains a statement about the functional intent of the exercises.

O: Veteran seen in room for AROM and strengthening of Ⓛ UE **in order to regain ability to dress self.** Pt. performed self-ranging exercises from standing and seated position with standby Ⓐ and verbal instructions to correct errors. Pt. was verbally cued x5 to reach higher with Ⓛ UE during shoulder flexion AROM.

Use Only Standard Abbreviations

You may use the abbreviations approved by your facility. For purposes of demonstration, a list of common abbreviations is provided in *Chapter Two: The Medical Record.* **Do not** use any other abbreviations, even if they seem common to you. If you try to read a note containing abbreviations with which you are unfamiliar, you will understand instantly how important this is. Remember that your documentation may be read by those unfamiliar with the "shorthand" that health professionals use so freely. Suppose your chart is being read by someone who is from a different background, such as an insurance clerk or an attorney or a committee at the Lion's Club who is considering funding a piece of adaptive equipment for your patient. To make your note understandable to all its readers, be judicious in applying abbreviations and keep them very standard.

Provide Complete Data in a Concise Format

In a **progress note,** you may be documenting test results. It is helpful to put the test results into a chart like the one below, rather than burying them in a narrative.

Sensory testing of Ⓛ hand revealed:
Hot/cold: intact
Sharp/dull: impaired over volar surface, intact over dorsal surface
Stereognosis: absent

The "O" section does not need to be written in complete sentences. Give complete information in the most concise form possible. Some details **must** be included. For example, ROM must be specified as active, passive or assistive and must indicate the joint at which the movement occurred. UE or LE must indicate which UE or LE. Level of assistance must be specified if assistance was given.

Being Specific About Assist Levels

When giving assist levels, be sure to note what part of the activity the patient needed assistance or verbal cues to perform. For example,

- Client doffed night garment with min Ⓐ **to untie strings on back.**
- Pt. required verbal cues **to sit down** in order to doff hosiery.
- Resident supine → sit in bed with minimal verbal cues **to roll to Ⓡ side.**
- Pt. stand → w/c using a standard walker with min physical Ⓐ and min verbal cues **to bring walker completely back to w/c.**
- Veteran washed upper body with min verbal cues **to initiate washing next part of body.**
- Standing pivot transfer with verbal cues **on hand placement needed for safety.**
- Client required mod Ⓐ **to follow total hip precautions** while using long-handled sponge for washing legs and feet.

When first learning to write the "O" section of the note, it is difficult to separate the objective data from the assessment data. Good OTAs automatically assess the data as they observe. In trying to separate "O" data from "A" data, some OTAs make the mistake of writing an "O" that contains only a list of actions with assist levels. While this is common, it is **incorrect**. Simply writing a list of activities or assist levels does not show skilled occupational therapy being provided. Consider this OTA's observation:

Pt. was seen for 1 hour in the shower room to ↑ activity tolerance and improve balance during showering, and was shown a smaller shower which simulated her home shower, in order to prepare for discharge in 1 week.

Pt. min Ⓐ with verbal cues to sit in w/c to doff hosiery and to dry off LE.

Pt. spontaneously rinsed soap off hands before gripping grab bar while showering.

Pt. used walker going to and coming from shower room.

Pt. tolerated standing Ⓘ during entire shower.

Pt. instructed in home showering.

Now let us look at the same observation, rewritten in a more useful format:

Pt. was seen for 1 hour in the shower room to ↑ activity tolerance and improve balance during showering and was also shown a smaller shower which simulated her home shower, in order to prepare her for Ⓘ and safe showering after discharge in 1 week.

Mobility: Pt walked to/from shower room Ⓘ and safely with the aid of a standard walker to provide stability in shower room while dressing/undressing.

Cognition: Pt. oriented x4.

ADL: Pt. min Ⓐ with verbal cues to sit down in order to towel dry LEs safely and to donn hosiery. During shower, pt. spontaneously rinsed soap off hands prior to gripping grab bar s̄ verbal cues. Pt. tolerated standing Ⓘ during shower s̄ SOB. Skilled instruction provided in safe technique to use in her single shower stall and recommendations given re: grab bar placement.

Worksheet 4-2

Being Specific About Assist Levels

When noting assist levels in your observation, it is not enough to note just the level of assistance required. You also need to note the part of the task that required assistance, for example:

Pt. donned pants with min Ⓐ to pull up over hips.

Pt. propelled w/c from room to occupational therapy clinic but required verbal cues to avoid running into other patients.

Assistance to sequence an activity is very different from assistance to maintain balance or to reach the feet while observing hip precautions.

Rewrite the statements below to provide a part of the task that required assistance. Since you have not seen the patient, you cannot know what part really required assistance. For this exercise, imagine a patient doing the task, then see what part of the task might have required assistance, and modify the sentences below accordingly.

1. Pt. supine → sit with min Ⓐ; bed → w/c with mod Ⓐ.

2. Pt. required SBA in transferring w/c → toilet.

3. Pt. retrieved garments from low drawers with min Ⓐ.

4. Brushing hair required max Ⓐ.

5. Pt. completed dressing, toileting, and hygiene with min Ⓐ.

De-Emphasizing the Treatment Media

In order to improve a patient's performance components you may utilize various media, such as equipment or activities that will help the patient reach functional goals. However, when documenting your observations of these treatment sessions, you should de-emphasize the media used, and focus instead on the performance components. For example, an OTA might write the following:

Patient worked on placing pegs into a pegboard.

This statement may accurately describe what a casual observer would see, but as a trained professional you need to look beyond the media used and see what the patient was really accomplishing. The media used here is pegs and a pegboard, but what is the performance component? Placing pegs into a pegboard is not a skill this patient needs in order to be able to care for herself, however, the performance component she practices during this activity may well be crucial to achieving independence. Suppose the therapist had written:

Patient worked on tripod pinch using pegs and a pegboard.

Notice that in this example the therapist did not simply add the performance component to the statement "Patient worked on placing pegs into a pegboard to increase tripod pinch" but actually turned the sentence around so that the tripod pinch received the emphasis and the media was mentioned only for clarification. Suppose that the therapist had written:

Patient worked on tripod pinch using pegs and a pegboard in order to be able to grasp objects needed for ADL tasks.

In this case, mention of the media becomes optional. She could also have written:

Patient worked on tripod pinch in order to be able to grasp objects needed for ADL tasks.

Which of the three preceding examples do you think best describes the skilled instruction that is occurring in this treatment session? This may seem like a minor distinction, but it is important in demonstrating the need for skilled occupational therapy and the emphasis on functional outcomes in therapy.

A common error among new OTAs is to focus on the media used, rather than on the performance component that is being improved by use of the media. Consider this OTA's observation:

Pt. was seen in rehab center for standing balance activities. Pt. stood to walker with min Ⓐ for balloon toss. Pt. used Ⓡ UE to hit balloon and was able to reach to Ⓡ and Ⓛ sides approximately 7 out of 10 tries. Activity was continued for 3 minutes. Pt. requested rest-break and sat for 30 seconds. Pt. then stood with mod Ⓐ to walker and hit balloon with Ⓛ UE for 3 minutes. Pt. was able to hit balloon approximately 6 out of 10 times and spontaneously switched to Ⓡ hand x2 when balloon was to her far right. Pt. sat for another break and to switch activities. Pt. stood CGA to toss beanbags with Ⓡ hand for 4 minutes. Pt. Scored 240 points with Ⓡ hand by throwing beanbags at target. Once all beanbags were thrown, pt. sat for a 30-second break. Pt. stood with CGA for balance to toss beanbags with Ⓛ hand for 30 seconds. Pt. scored 150 points with Ⓛ hand by throwing beanbags at scoring target. Once all beanbags were thrown, pt. sat and session was ended.

When this note is rewritten to focus on the performance components, notice the difference in professionalism in the way the note reads:

Pt. seen in clinic for dynamic and static standing balance activities. Pt stood to walker with min Ⓐ for dynamic standing balance necessary for Ⓘ showering using a balloon toss activity. Pt. held walker with Ⓛ hand and used Ⓡ UE to reach both Ⓡ and Ⓛ sides approximately 7/10 attempts. Pt. sustained activity for 3 minutes continuously and then took a 30-second rest break. Pt. stood to walker again with mod Ⓐ for 3 minutes of continuous activity involving weight shifting and balance required in balloon tossing. Pt. demonstrated ability to reach to Ⓡ and Ⓛ sides to reach for moving object approximately 6/10 times. Pt. demonstrated ability to spontaneously shift weight 2 times to reach object. Pt. took 30-second rest break before next activity. Pt. worked on dynamic standing balance using beanbag toss activity with target. Pt. stood to walker for 4 minutes of dynamic balance activity with CGA, then sat for 30-second rest. Pt. stood again with CGA for 3 ½ minutes of dynamic balance activity.

In mental health settings, it is particularly important to focus on the purpose of the activity if a craft project or other creative media is being used. For example, you may be using a creative project to facilitate self-esteem, to encourage self-expression, or to evaluate the ability to follow instructions. These performance components should be the focus of your note, rather than the project that was used. For example, the following note describes the projects used by an OTA during a treatment session in a mental health clinic:

Patient seen for 45 minutes to work on leather project. He worked for 10 minutes, then got one of the loops in his stitches turned around wrong, put down his key case, looked out the window, and frowned until the OTA asked him what was wrong and helped him correct the error he had made. He did not make any eye contact with the OTA or the group members, and did not participate in conversation with others in the group. When cued to resume work, he started stitching again, using a single cordovan stitch, did so for 5 more minutes, until he got another stitch turned over wrong. Twice during the session he was able to correct his own errors. He never did ask for help, but again frowned and looked out the window until the OTA noticed he needed some help, got the error corrected, showed him the correct way to make the stitch, and reminded him to get back to work. He never did talk to anyone, or even make any eye contact. After his last error 20 minutes into the session, he put his head on the table and kept it there the rest of the session, refusing to do any more stitches on his project, or talk to the other patients in the group.

This note would provide better documentation on the performance components addressed during the occupational therapy treatment if it were written as follows:

Patient seen for 45-minute activity group to work on attention span, social skills, and successful leisure experiences. Pt. worked on task for a maximum of 20 minutes before placing head on table and declining further activity. Patient able to correct 2 errors independently, but put down project and looked out of the window while frowning 3x rather than request help when other errors were made. Verbal cues needed to resume activity after errors were corrected. Pt. made no eye contact and did not interact with peers (Mason, 2001).

Worksheet 4-3

De-Emphasizing the Treatment Media

Rewrite the following statements to emphasize the skilled occupational therapy that is actually occurring in the treatment session:

1. Patient played pegboard game to work on functional grasp.

2. Patient played catch using bilateral UEs to facilitate grasp and release pattern.

3. Patient put dirt into pot to ½ way point, added seedling, and filled remainder of pot with dirt transferred by cup. Pt. completed 3 more pots while standing 8 minutes before requiring a 5-minute rest. Pt. resumed standing position to water completed pots for approximately 5 minutes.

Being Concise in Your Wording

When first learning to write patient observations, it is hard to decide what to include and what to leave out. At first, it is best to include too much data, rather than take a chance on omitting something important. As your observational skills become more refined, it will become second nature to include all the important data, and the "O" section of your notes will begin to be more concise. Here is a patient observation written by an inexperienced therapist. In an effort to include all the necessary data she wrote a note that was too "wordy".

> *Pt. was seen in therapy room for Ⓡ UE strengthening. Pt. was asked to clasp hands together and raise arms above head 30x. Pt was then instructed to cross her midline and touch her opposite shoulder with Ⓡ UE. Pt. required 6 rest periods for completion. Pt. completed tasks Ⓘ. Pt. was then introduced to weight and pulley system. Pt. was asked to specify how much weight she thought she could do. She responded with 5#. Pt. did 30 reps of the pulley system with 5# in shoulder flexion to strengthen her rotator cuff to decrease the probability of dislocating her shoulder again. After strengthening exercise pt. had 3 heat packs applied to shoulder to decrease pain.*

A more experienced therapist might have written:

> *Pt. seen in clinic for the following Ⓡ UE strengthening exercises for rotator cuff in order to prevent further dislocation:*
>
> *Ⓑ clasped hand shoulder flexion and extension x 30 repetitions*
>
> *Horizontal adduction Ⓡ hand to Ⓛ shoulder x 30 repetitions*
>
> *Ⓡ shoulder flexion pulleys with 5# wt. x 30 repetitions*
>
> *3 hot packs used to ↓ pain after treatment*

You will notice, however, that there is another problem with this note besides the fact that it is "wordy". It also sounds like a physical therapy note rather than an occupational therapy note. This note needs to have functional components added, although they do not have to be in the "O." A statement from the patient in the "S" about what she is unable to do with an injured rotator cuff and a statement in the "A" and/or "P" indicating functional problems/goals would suffice to make it a good occupational therapy note. Notice that being more concise means knowing what information can be omitted without compromising the quality of the observation.

Worksheet 4-4

Being Concise

Now it's your turn. Reword the following note to be more concise:

O: Pt seen bedside. Pt. ambulated ~36 inches to shower with SBA for safety. Pt. instructed to complete shower while sitting. Pt. performed shower with SBA to manage IV line. Pt. able to wash upper and lower body Ⓘ and dry entire body after completing shower. Pt. required ~20 minutes to complete shower. Pt. then ambulated ~36 inches to chair and sat. Pt. needed verbal cues to remain seated while donning underwear and pants. Pt. able to dress UE Ⓘ and lower body $\overline{p}$ verbal cues for sitting. Pt. demonstrated good sitting balance, but needed SBA for standing balance. Following shower, pt. stated he would like to take a nap and was assisted back into bed.

Avoid Being Judgmental in Your Wording

When you are working with a patient who is difficult, or who has opinions and behavior with which you do not agree, it is easy to judge the patient and to reflect your judgments in your observation. Below is a note written by a student who was in a difficult situation. The patient "went off on" the student, refusing a sponge bath, lying about having already bathed, throwing her washcloth across the room so that the student would have to pick it up, refusing to put on her slacks, and announcing that therapy was "stupid." In spite of all this, the student wrote an observation that was non-judgmental of the patient:

> *Pt. required max encouragement to participate in therapy this AM. Pt. Ⓘ sit → stand & ambulating to sink. Pt. Ⓘ at sink c̄ simulated bathing activity using long handled sponge. Pt. Ⓘ retrieved washcloth from floor using a reacher. Pt. Ⓘ set-up to don/doff shoes and socks using adaptive equipment. Pt. retrieved gown and socks Ⓘ with a reacher. Pt. declined to don slacks.*

Helpful Hint

Good documentation is based on accurate observation, which is based on knowing what to look for. For an experienced therapist, this becomes second nature. For a student therapist, it is helpful to review the lists in this manual and to check your observations against what your supervising therapist observed during the treatment session to be sure you are noticing the items that matter most.

Chapter Five

Writing the "A" – Assessment

The third section of the note is the **ASSESSMENT**, which contains the therapist's opinion or judgment regarding the client's progress, functional limitations, and expected benefit from rehabilitation. In the assessment section of the note, you will interpret the meaning of the data you have presented in the "O" portion of your note, describing what it means in your professional judgment, and its potential impact on the patient's occupational performance.

For example, during the treatment session, you may have observed that the patient falls over to the left when he tries to sit unsupported at the edge of his bed. You will note both the problem (static sitting balance) and the performance areas in which it is a problem (transfers and basic ADL tasks). In your assessment, you might say something like:

Lack of static sitting balance raises safety concerns when patient transfers w/c to bed or toilet, and when sitting EOB for basic hygiene and dressing tasks.

In the assessment section of your note, you will primarily note the three P's: problems, progress, and rehab potential. You might also point out inconsistencies, discuss emotional components, or present some reason that something was not done as planned.

Assessing the Data

To assess the data, go **sentence by sentence** through the data presented in the "S" and the "O," asking yourself what it means for the patient's occupational performance. Note what problems, progress, or potential for rehabilitation you see. Consider some of the following possibilities:

Problems may include some of the following:

Safety risks.

- Safety concerns noted when patient attempted to stand without locking brakes on w/c.
- Poor problem-solving when using the stove raises safety concerns.
- Client's limited coping strategies for dealing with stress raise concerns for continuing the use of self-destructive behaviors.

Inconsistencies between patient report and objective findings:

- Although patient anticipates no difficulty in returning to pre-hospitalization level of home-making activity, her left-side neglect could cause significant in-home safety risks.
- Although the patient expresses a willingness to do ADL tasks, motor planning problems create a barrier to the task.
- Client verbalizes a desire to progress to the next level of responsibility, but shows ↓ behavioral control when reward incentives are unavailable.

Areas of performance not WFL that can be influenced by OT intervention, for example:

- Left-side weakness interferes with standing balance in tub.
- Left-side neglect necessitates verbal cues to complete ADL tasks.
- Due to deficits in cognitive processing, patient currently needs constant verbal cues to perform kitchen tasks safely.
- Lack of forearm supination limits Katie's ability to engage in developmental play activities.
- Lack of spatial orientation to identify letter shapes interferes with ability to learn to read.
- Child's delayed visual motor skills for chronological age affects ability to perform kindergarten tasks.

Emotional or mental health components:

- Continued verbal threats toward other patients indicate a need for anger management techniques.
- Molly's continued isolation of herself in her room rather than attending groups interferes with learning to interact with unfamiliar people and situations.

Progress or indications that the treatment being provided is effective:

- Weighted utensils decrease intention tremors by ~50%.
- Patient has gained 10 degrees AROM in the left elbow this week.
- Patient has made gains since 11/17/01 by demonstrating the ability to follow 1-step commands 80% of the time.
- Jack is making progress toward re-entry into the community as shown by his ability to prepare for an outing, respect rules by following directions, interact socially with staff, and control his behavior.
- Client's spontaneous participation in group discussion shows that he is making progress in developing social interaction skills.
- UE strength is increasing as demonstrated by ability to pull to stand.
- Child's progress from 70% to 90% accuracy in shape recognition indicates good recall.

Sometimes you will need to explain the lack of progress:

- Patient has become more dependent in ADL tasks this week due to acute infection.

Sometimes progress is indicated by stating that previous goals have been met or changed:

- STG #2 (buttoning ½ inch buttons x3 on shirt) met this week.
- STG #4 changed to "greet other patients when entering room".

Potential for success in rehabilitation:

- Ability to understand instructions and desire to return to living independently indicate good rehab potential.
- Patient's ability to recall and demonstrate 3/3 hip precautions shows good potential to return to prior living situation.
- Patient's intact manipulative skills and fine motor coordination make him a good candidate for rehabilitation.
- Child's progress from 60% to 70% accuracy of reproducing shapes indicates good potential to meet goals stated in IEP.
- Client's ability to recognize stressors shows good potential to change self-destructive coping strategies.
- Participation in groups, including not interrupting, asking questions appropriately, and sharing experiences indicate good potential to benefit from psychiatric rehab program.

Writing the Assessment

Identifying Significant Areas

As you read carefully through the material in your "S" and your "O", it is sometimes helpful to make a quick list of things you want to discuss in the "A" section of your note. For example, consider the following "S" and "O":

S: Client stated that he gets bored during the day when he has nothing to do, and said "I wish I had a car so I could get out easier."

O: Client seen in his home and taken on city bus for community re-integration following discharge from inpatient facility. Client demonstrated home management skills and ability to care for animals by simulation. Client was able to identify which bus to catch to go to grocery store, but needed reassurance that his choice was correct. At the grocery store, client chose lunchmeat and fruit for lunches this week, but needed SBA for payment.

This therapist identified the following areas of progress, problems, and potential.

PROGRESS

- Client is able to simulate care of home and animals.
- Client is able to choose the correct bus to get to the grocery store.
- Client is willing to choose healthier foods at the store this visit.

PROBLEMS

- Client is anxious about whether his bus choice is really correct.
- Client is still unable to manage money independently.

POTENTIAL

In her professional judgment, the progress shown to date is also a good indicator of rehab potential for this patient. She writes her assessment of the data as follows:

A: Client's ability to demonstrate home and animal care activities as taught earlier shows good progress toward being able to live independently in the community. Client also demonstrates progress in community mobility by being able to identify which bus to take to the grocery store this visit, and in ability to care for self by choosing healthier foods rather than his former choices of chips and donuts. Anxiety level in selecting the correct bus and need for assistance in managing money continue to limit client's functional independence.

New Information

The assessment section is **not** the place to introduce new data. Do not put anything in your "A" that has not been discussed in "O." If you find yourself wanting to make a statement in the "A" that is not supported by the data in your "O", ask yourself what you might have observed to support the assessment statement. Then decide whether you need to add it to your "O."

Justifying Continued Treatment

One very useful way of justifying continued OT treatment for your patient is to end the "A" with the statement "Patient would benefit from..." and complete the sentence with a justification of continued treatment that requires the skill of an OT or OTA, based on your observations and assessment. Not every therapist ends the "A" in this fashion, but for purposes of learning we will end the "A" in this way. This helps to make certain that justification for continued treatment is present in the note, and is a good method of setting up the plan. After you are more proficient in writing notes and are certain that your note justifies continued treatment, you may choose to cover this material in the plan instead. Below are some examples:

- Resident would benefit from environmental cues to orient him to environment.
- Patient would benefit from further ADL training along with visual perceptual and problem-solving activities.
- Veteran would benefit from activities that encourage trunk rotation to facilitate transfers and dressing skills.
- Patient would benefit from continued mental health education including recognition of his delusions, need for medication, how it can help him, and why it is essential to his recovery.
- Jim would benefit from compensatory techniques to differentiate letter shapes needed to progress in reading skills.
- Patient would benefit from reacher, sock aid, and long-handled shoe horn to aid in lower body dressing.
- Resident would benefit from skilled instruction in sequencing of tasks to increase safety while performing ADL tasks.
- Patient would benefit from instruction in energy conservation techniques to perform meal preparation and cleanup.
- Client would benefit from continued use of modalities which ↓ sensory defensiveness.
- JW would benefit from continued instruction in problem-solving and anger management techniques needed for successful personal and social relationships.

Ending the Assessment

Now we can finish the assessment section of the note we began earlier:

S: Client stated that he gets bored during the day when he has nothing to do, and said "I wish I had a car so I could get out easier."

O: Client seen in his home and taken on city bus for community re-integration following discharge from inpatient facility. Client demonstrated ability to care for home and animals by simulation. Client able to identify which bus to catch to go to grocery store, but needed reassurance that his choice was correct. At the grocery store, client chose lunchmeat and fruit for lunches this week, but needed SBA for payment.

A: Client's ability to demonstrate home and animal care activities as taught earlier shows good progress toward being able to live independently in the community. Client also demonstrates progress in community mobility by being able to identify which bus to take to the grocery store this visit, and in ability to care for self by choosing healthier foods than his former choices of chips and donuts. Anxiety level in selecting the correct bus and need for assistance in managing money continue to limit client's functional independence. Client would benefit from continued instruction in going to new places in the community and instruction in money management to increase his ability to shop without caregiver support.

The following are examples of what the completed assessment section of your note might look like:

A: Inability to don prosthesis Ⓘ currently limits Ⓘ in ambulation needed for functional toileting. Pt. would benefit from additional skilled instruction and practice in use of pulley-like fasteners on prosthesis to allow one-handed closure installed this date.

A: Martha is beginning to regain some of the independent living skills she had prior to her recent psychotic episode. Fear, isolation, and ↓ activity tolerance slow her progress and are the focus of current treatment. Martha would benefit from continued skilled instruction in self-care skills as well as ↑ socialization and ↑ physical activity.

A: Mary's use of her left hand as a functional assist 60% of the time continues to limit her independence in self-care and play tasks. She would benefit from more bilateral activities to ↑ use of left hand during play.

A: Patient's spontaneous actions in groups, willingness to share verbally, and improved dress and hygiene seem to indicate an improved mood this week. Progress also noted in unprompted attendance, which is up this week, from 2/8 to 6/8 groups attended. Goals #1 (assertion) and #2 (communication) are met as of this date. Goal #3 (leisure skills) is continued through discharge, pending formulation of a plan for use of leisure time.

In addition, it is necessary to document the reason the service must be provided by an OT or OTA rather than by another professional or by nonprofessional personnel.

Occupational therapists provide the following services:

- Evaluate patients, identify problems, establish goals, and develop treatment plans.
- Assess or reassess the effectiveness of adaptive equipment/techniques.

Occupational therapists and occupational therapy assistants provide the following services:

- Modify functional tasks/activities, modify homes or other environmental contexts.
- Modify activities through the use of adaptive equipment/assistive devices.
- Provide and instruct in the use of adaptive equipment; instruct in adaptive techniques.
- Fabricate splints and adaptive devices.
- Provide individualized instruction to the patient/family/caregiver.
- Determine that the procedure/equipment used is safe and effective.
- Intervene to prevent safety hazards and unsafe behaviors.
- Teach compensatory skills.
- Improve performance areas through remediation.

- Instruct in energy conservation and work simplification.
- Instruct in joint protection (Cullen, 1998).

Skilled occupational therapy is **not** evident when the OT or OTA provides the following services:

- Continues treatment after goals are reached or no further significant progress is expected.
- Carries out a maintenance program.
- Provides routine strengthening or exercise programs if there is no potential for functional improvement.
- Carries out daily programs after the adapted procedures are in place and no further progress is expected.
- Presents information such as handouts on energy conservation without having the patient or caregiver perform the activity.
- Provides service to a patient who has poor rehabilitation potential.
- Duplicates services with another discipline (Cullen, 1998).

Wording is critical to documenting the necessity for continuing skilled occupational therapy. Under the supervision of an OT, the OTA provides skilled instruction to patients rather than assisting them. For example, an OTA may provide training in methods of energy conservation and work simplification instead of helping the patient to perform a strenuous task. An OTA may provide instruction and training in home programs, which will be carried out by aides and family members.

Why should a third party payer reimburse you to watch a patient carry out a home exercise program that he performs daily on his own? If you determine a patient is not performing all components of the program correctly and you alter the program to address the recent problems, then your professional skill in modifying the program is clearly required. Analyze your clinical reasoning and then document the principles and strategies used during a treatment session in justifying the continuation of skilled occupational therapy.

Remember that the justification for continued treatment must support the frequency and duration of the plan. If the last sentence of your "A" reads: "Patient would benefit from information on energy conservation techniques", do not expect the payer to approve more than one more treatment session.

HELPFUL HINT

Assessment is the "heart" of your note. If you could write only six lines, the assessment section of your note would contain the six lines you would choose. This is the section that demonstrates your clinical reasoning as an OTA.

Worksheet 5-1

Justifying Continued Treatment

Which of the following require the skill of an OTA?

_____ The practice of coordination and self-care skills on a daily basis.

_____ Modifying functional tasks/activities through the provision of adaptive equipment or techniques.

_____ Determining that the modified task is safe and effective.

_____ Carrying out a maintenance program.

_____ Teaching the patient to use the breathing techniques he has been taught while performing his ADL activities.

_____ Providing individualized instruction to the patient, family, or caregiver.

_____ Provision of specialized instruction to eliminate limitations in a functional activity.

_____ Instructing caregivers.

_____ Making changes in the environment.

_____ Teaching compensatory skills.

_____ Gait training.

_____ Intervening with patients to eliminate safety hazards.

_____ Presenting information handouts (such as energy conservation) without having the patient perform the activity.

_____ Routine exercise and strengthening programs.

_____ Adding instruction in lower body dressing techniques to a current ADL program.

_____ Teaching adaptive techniques such as one-handed shoe tying.

_____ Advancing a treatment plan that is in place.

Worksheet 5-2

Assessing the "Categories" Note

In *Chapter Three: Writing the "S"—Subjective,* the following observation was used as a demonstration. Now we will look at its content more carefully, and draw some conclusions about its content.

The "Categories" Observation

S: Patient says she is unable to move right UE, although she does not know why it will not move. She reports "It really doesn't hurt. It's just tight."

O: Patient seen in rehab gym for UE activities to ↑ AROM in Ⓡ shoulder, activity tolerance, UE strength, and dynamic standing balance, in order to ↑ independence in ADL activities.

ADL: Pt. seen in room for instruction in safety techniques and adaptive equipment use in toileting. Pt. needs bilateral grab bars in bathroom to sit → stand safely. Patient attempted to stand while pulling on walker and one grab bar. Patient was instructed on safety issues and the use of bilateral grab bars.

Performance components: Pt. sit → stand CGA for balance. Pt. worked on activity tolerance, dynamic standing balance and ↓ AROM in right shoulder by moving canned goods from counter to cupboard for 5 minutes before needing a 2-minute sitting rest. After resting, participated in activities to ↑ dynamic standing balance by pouring liquid from a pitcher while standing CGA for balance. After a 1-minute rest, pt. continued activities to dynamic standing balance and safety in ADL activities by pushing wheeled walker while picking up objects from the floor with a reacher. AROM in right shoulder abduction <90°. PROM right shoulder abduction WNL.

How would you assess this information? Go back and look at the suggestions given earlier in the chapter. What problems can you identify? Do you see evidence of progress? Safety risks? Performance areas not WFL that occupational therapy might impact? Is there any indication of the patient's rehab potential? What would this patient benefit from?

After you identify problems, progress, and rehab potential, write below your assessment based on the information above.

A:

In preparing an assessment of the data in this note, this OTA assesses two main **problem** areas: the safety of transferring to and from the toilet, and the performance components that were not WFL. This OTA was particularly concerned about the safety issues, and addressed those first. She also noted the rehabilitation **potential** that would be helpful to a reviewer in deciding whether the patient's progress is sufficient to warrant the expense of treatment.

A: Safety concerns (impulsivity, ↓ dynamic standing balance) noted when patient attempts to transfer sit → stand during toileting. Pt. verbalized an understanding of safety instructions and has potential to progress to independence.

Next she addressed the clinical reasoning behind devoting time to addressing performance components with this patient, in the light of his rehab potential.

A: Safety concerns (impulsivity, ↓ dynamic standing balance) noted when patient attempts to transfer sit → stand during toileting. Pt. verbalized an understanding of safety instructions and has potential to progress to independence. Pt.'s ↓ AROM in right shoulder, ↓ activity tolerance, and ↓ dynamic standing balance all interfere with ability to complete ADL tasks safely and independently.

She completes the assessment by justifying continued treatment

A: Safety concerns (impulsivity, ↓ dynamic standing balance) noted when patient attempts to transfer sit → stand during toileting. Pt. verbalized an understanding of safety instructions and has potential to progress to independence. Pt.'s ↓ AROM in right shoulder, ↓ activity tolerance, and ↓ dynamic standing balance all interfere with ability to complete ADL tasks safely and independently. Pt. would benefit from Ⓡ UE AROM and strengthening exercises along with continued skilled instruction in safety issues and energy conservation techniques.

In *Chapter Six: Writing the "P" — Plan* you will see how this OTA plans to provide the things this patient would benefit from in a cost-effective manner. You will also be writing several more assessments in the next chapter, along with a plan to carry out the treatment from which you have suggested the patient would benefit.

Assessing Problems Not Within Functional Limits

Some notes will show **progress** and/or rehab **potential**, and some will not, but almost all notes will show **problem** areas, because the problems are what keep a patient in active treatment. The most common problem area that you will be assessing is the impact of a performance component that is not within functional limits (WFL). When students are first learning to write SOAP notes, they may find it difficult to distinguish observations from assessments. There is a formula you can use to write about a problem area that is not WFL, ensuring that you are writing an assessment rather than an observation. This formula calls for making the performance component the subject of the sentence, and then telling how that performance component impacts a patient's functional ability in a particular performance area.

Performance Component	Impact	Performance Area

For example:

- Deficits in UE strength and activity tolerance limit patient's ability to complete basic self-care tasks.
- Lack of forearm supination and active elbow flexion against gravity interfere with child's ability to perform age-appropriate developmental play activities.
- Pain in Ⓛ shoulder limits patient's ability to carry out child-care and household management tasks.
- Deficits in attention span make instrumental ADLs difficult and possibly unsafe.
- Inability to manage anger results in difficulty finding work and establishing successful intimate relationships.
- Decreased strength and AROM interfere with patient's ability to transfer and to propel w/c Ⓘ.

Notice that in each of the examples given above, the performance component that is not WFL is the subject of the sentence, and then is followed by the negative impact it has on a specific performance area. This is not the only way to write assessment statements, but the formula given is a good one to use when you are first learning.

Worksheet 5-3

Assessing Problems Not Within Functional Limits

You will be rewriting some assessment statements to make them more effective using the following formula:

Performance Component	Impact	Performance Area

For example, the statement:

Patient's activity tolerance for lower body dressing was <2 minutes secondary to SOB from asthma.

does have the information it needs, but would be more effective if written by the formula above. Using the formula you might write:

Patient's SOB and activity tolerance of 2 minutes is insufficient for dressing her lower body.

Re-write the following statements using the formula given above:

1. Patient demonstrated difficulty with laundry and cooking tasks due to memory and sequencing deficits.

2. Decreased level of arousal noted during morning dressing activities, requiring redirection to task.

3. Patient unable to follow hip precautions during morning dressing due to memory deficits.

4. Patient problem-solved poorly while performing lower body dressing as evidenced by multiple attempts to button pants and don socks.

Worksheet 5-4

Assessing a Note

Now it is time to practice what you have learned. Here are the "S" and "O" sections of a note.

S: When asked, pt. stated that he had rested well and was ready to work.

O: Pt. seen bedside in order to work on trunk stability, midline crossing, and bilateral integration in order to improve performance of basic ADLs.

Posture and balance: Pt's posture appears slightly asymmetrical in that he laterally flexes to left & bears weight mostly on Ⓡ hip. Head turned slightly to Ⓡ; shoulders are asymmetrical; Ⓛ shoulder is elevated and protracted.
Vision: Pt's visual perceptual skills appear WFL.
Following commands and expression: Pt. able to follow verbal commands 100% of the time and he displays appropriate affect during conversation 100% of the time.
Movement: When asked to reach forward with Ⓛ UE, pt. used compensatory technique of elevating shoulder and laterally flexing to Ⓡ. While midline crossing to Ⓛ, pt. required verbal cues to shift weight to left and to incorporate Ⓛ UE. Pt. required muscle tapping in order to depress Ⓛ shoulder during reach patterns.
Transfers and dressing: Pt. required max Ⓐ for trunk stability in transfer bed → w/c and needed max Ⓐ in dressing due to ↓ AROM of Ⓛ UE and poor trunk mobility.

First, make a list of the problems, progress, or rehab potential that you notice in the observation. For any problem you identify, note the performance area that is affected.

- Problems (and performance area affected):

- Progress (if any):

- Rehab Potential:

Next, write an assessment of the observation, based on the items you have listed.

A:

Chapter Six

Writing the "P"— Plan

The last section of a SOAP note is the **PLAN** where the OTA sets forth the specific treatment that the patient will receive to achieve the goals. The plan should relate to the information presented in the assessment. It will inform the reader what you plan to do next in treatment. In this book, you will learn to end the "P" with a goal. This is not the only correct way to write a plan, but it is the one we will be using. Usually a short-term goal is used. The choice of what kind of goal to use depends on the facility. In a long-term care facility where notes are written monthly, your goal would be what you hope to accomplish in the next month. In an acute care setting, it would be your goal for tomorrow. In some settings, the "A" section of the SOAP note will specify what goals were met and will also set new goals.

The OT who initially evaluated the patient will estimate the frequency and duration of treatment that will be needed to accomplish the goals. This estimate, based on typical or established timelines for specific diagnoses, will be included in the treatment plan of the initial evaluation. In the "P" of progress notes, you will address how often you will see the patient, how long treatment will continue, and set your priorities for what you will work on next. You will end this section with either your long-term goal or your short-term goal, whichever is appropriate to your treatment setting. (Usually the short-term goal is used.) Goals are always written in measurable, objective, behavioral terms, and include a function and a time line. For example:

Pt. will ____________________ ____________________ ____________________
(action verb) (skill) (under what conditions)

______________________________ ______________.
(for what function—if not already indicated) (by when)

Examples of a "P" might include:

- Resident to be seen for 2 more weeks for ½ hr. b.i.d. sessions for skilled instruction in meal/snack preparation and clean-up. By discharge on 8/13/01, resident will be able to prepare a TV dinner in the microwave Ⓘ at wheelchair level.
- Continue 1 hour daily sessions for 1 week. Within 1 week, veteran will demonstrate the ability to put arms in holes of shirt 50% of the time after set up and <3 verbal cues.
- Child will continue to be seen 2x wk for ½ hour sessions in order to ↑ fine motor skills for better classroom performance within 2 weeks. Child will be able to cut a curved line Ⓘ within ¼ inch 3/3 tries by 2/4/01.
- Pt. will continue to be seen in groups 5x wk for 1 week to work on assertion skills and anger management. Pt. will attend 75% of groups without prompting and will spontaneously participate in discussion >5 times by 4/2/01.
- Consumer will continue sheltered workshop program 5 days/wk in order to ↑ work skills. Consumer will attend to task for 60 minutes with no verbal cues within 1 week in order to ↑ Ⓘ as a worker.

HELPFUL HINT

If for some reason you are not able to see your patient as scheduled, the "P" section of your note should allow another therapist to continue treatment uninterrupted.

Planning for the Categories Note

Now let us write a plan for the "Categories" note we assessed in the last chapter.

S: Patient says she is unable to move right UE, although she does not know why it will not move. She reports "It really doesn't hurt. It's just tight."

O: Patient seen in rehab gym for UE activities to ↑ AROM in Ⓡ shoulder, activity tolerance, UE strength, and dynamic standing balance in order to ↑ independence in ADL activities.

ADL: Pt. seen in room for instruction in safety techniques and adaptive equipment use in toileting. Pt. needs bilateral grab bars in bathroom to sit → stand safely. Patient attempted to stand while pulling on walker and one grab bar. Patient was instructed on safety issues and the use of bilateral grab bars.

Performance components: Pt. sit → stand CGA for balance. Pt. worked on activity tolerance, dynamic standing balance and ↑ AROM in Ⓡ shoulder by moving canned goods from counter to cupboard for 5 minutes before needing a 2 minute sitting rest. After resting, participated in activities to ↑ dynamic standing balance by pouring liquid from a pitcher while standing CGA for balance. After a 1-minute rest, pt. continued activities to ↑ dynamic standing balance and safety in ADL activities by pushing wheeled walker while picking up objects from the floor with a reacher. AROM in right shoulder abduction <90°. PROM right shoulder abduction WNL.

A: Safety concerns (impulsivity, ↓ dynamic standing balance) noted when patient attempts to transfer sit → stand during toileting. Pt. verbalized an understanding of safety instructions and has potential to progress to independence. Pt.'s ↓ AROM in right shoulder, ↓ activity tolerance, and ↓ dynamic standing balance all interfere with ability to complete ADL tasks safely and independently. Pt. would benefit from UE AROM and strengthening exercises along with continued skilled instruction in safety issues and energy conservation techniques.

Write your plan for this patient below. Begin with a statement about how often (b.i.d., daily, 2x wk, etc.) and for how long (for 3 days, for 2 weeks, for 1 month, etc.) she will be treated. Look at the items above that she would benefit from, and set your priorities. End with a correctly written goal.

Worksheet 6-1

Final SOAP Note for a Treatment Session Written in "Categories"

P:

Completing the Plan for the Categories Note

In assessing the data, the OTA has set up the plan for this note. She has already justified the main things she intended to do and indicated the patient's rehabilitation potential. Now she needs to be specific about how often the patient will be treated and for what length of time. She first specifies the frequency and duration of treatment.

P: Continue to treat patient 5x wk for 1 week.

She could have specified the length of the treatment sessions, i.e., *for 1 hr. sessions*, but this therapist chose not to do that in this particular note. Next she specifies how she plans to use the treatment time:

P: Continue to treat patient 5x wk for 1 week for skilled instruction in safe transfers and toileting.

Since she anticipates discharge in one week, she has to prioritize her time. She chooses to work on balance and energy conservation as a part of functional mobility and ADL activities. Since she has already written that the patient would benefit from additional AROM and strengthening exercises, she now needs to specify how she plans to address this need.

P: Continue to treat patient 5x wk for 1 week for skilled instruction in safe transfers and toileting. Home program for AROM and strengthening exercises for Ⓡ shoulder will be taught.

This OTA has also indicated clinical reasoning in planning for discharge in advance of the discharge date. In later notes she will indicate the patient's progress in learning the home program. Simply handing the patient a set of printed exercises is not considered a billable service. The patient's progress in learning the home program will also confirm the OTA's assessment that the patient's rehabilitation potential was on target. She will end this plan with a measurable, action oriented, time-limited goal. Notice that she has specified the conditions under which this action will be carried out.

P: Continue to treat patient 5x wk for 1 week to work on safe transfers and toileting. Home program for AROM and strengthening exercises for Ⓡ shoulder will be taught. Pt. will demonstrate ability to transfer to toilet safely with CGA and use of walker and grab bars by the end of 5 tx sessions.

This note is now complete.

Some therapists provide each short-term goal with a number. For example:

STG #1: Resident will prepare a TV dinner in the microwave Ⓘ at w/c level by discharge on 8/13/01.

STG #2: Resident will clear his place setting and wash dishes Ⓘ by 8/13/01.

In notes to follow, the therapist can refer to those numbered goals, providing a clear indication of the progress achieved. For example:

A: STG #1: met. STG #2: Res. requires min Ⓐ to maneuver w/c around table in kitchen and place w/c in appropriate location to reach sink, wash dishes and put away in cabinets while seated in w/c.

P: Resident will continue to be treated until d/c in 1 week. At time of d/c res. will be Ⓘ in all meal prep and clean-up while seated in w/c.

Worksheet 6-2

Completing the Plan for the Postural Instability Note

Now it is your turn. In the last chapter, you wrote an assessment for a treatment note on postural instability. Now you will have the opportunity to complete that note by adding a plan.

S: When asked, pt. stated that he had rested well and was ready to work.

O: Pt. seen bedside in order to work on trunk stability, midline crossing, and bilateral integration in order to improve performance of basic ADLs.

Posture and balance: Pt.'s posture appears slightly asymmetrical in that he laterally flexes to left & bears weight mostly on Ⓡ hip. Head turned slightly to Ⓡ; shoulders are asymmetrical; Ⓛ shoulder is elevated and protracted.

Vision: Pt.'s visual perceptual skills appear WFL.

Following commands and expression: Pt. able to follow verbal commands 100% of the time and he displays appropriate affect during conversation 100% of the time.

Movement: When asked to reach forward with Ⓛ UE, pt. used compensatory technique of elevating shoulder and laterally flexing to Ⓡ. While midline crossing to Ⓛ, pt. required verbal cues to shift weight to left and to incorporate Ⓛ UE. Pt. required muscle tapping in order to depress Ⓛ shoulder during reach patterns.

Transfers and dressing: Pt. required max Ⓐ for trunk stability in transfer bed → w/c and needed max Ⓐ in dressing due to ↓ AROM of Ⓛ UE and poor trunk mobility.

A: Decreased trunk stability causes asymmetrical posture, which results in safety concerns during transfers. Decreased AROM in the Ⓛ UE results in decreased bilateral integration and midline crossing which decreases the patient's ability to perform basic ADL tasks. Ability to follow directions 100% of the time and good visual perceptual skills indicate good rehab potential. Patient would benefit from continued activities to increase trunk stability and AROM of the Ⓛ UE needed for dressing and transfers.

Write your plan for this note below:

P:

Worksheet 6-3

The Exercise Note

For the next two exercises, we will do the "A" and "P" sections as a unit. Read the following observation of a treatment session and formulate an assessment and a plan based on the information provided. Although we will "walk through" this note together on the next page, please do not read ahead to find out how the writer words the "A" and "P" sections. It is far more effective to practice your skill at writing assessments and plans before finding out how someone else might have written the same information.

Observation of a Treatment Session Primarily Devoted to Exercise

S: Pt. reports being pleased with her progress in functional mobility since last tx session.

O: Pt. was seen in OT clinic to work on bilateral UE strengthening and AROM in order to improve bilateral UE function in ADLs. She required min Ⓐ with w/c mobility room → clinic, requiring verbal instructions not to hit the wall and an occasional push when she lost momentum. Pt. then completed Ⓛ UE strengthening exercises using yellow theraband:

elbow flexion x15
elbow extension x15

Pt. then completed Ⓡ UE strengthening and AROM with the following results:

right forearm: pronation: full AROM supination: ½ AROM
right wrist: extension: ½ AROM (x10 repetitions)
radial and ulnar deviation: WFL
fingers: flexion and extension: full AROM
thumb: opposition: full AROM

Pt. was able to demonstrate isolated 3+ finger flexion and extension in all 5 digits. Brunnstrom arm exercises with AAROM to Ⓡ UE to increase strength and AROM for donning shirt using over-the-head method. Results: (bilateral shoulder)

elevation/depression x5
flexion x5
horizontal ab/adduction x5

A:

P:

Assessing and Planning for the Exercise Note

When a treatment session is devoted primarily to addressing performance components, it is critical to tie the performance components back into function. This note addresses function in some manner in all four sections, even though the treatment session was devoted to exercise. Note that in the observation, the therapist specified that the exercises were for the purpose of improving UE function in ADL tasks. In the assessment she will reiterate that she is basically trying to improve function in ADL tasks by working on the underlying factors that prevent independent functioning.

Having reported the basic measurements and assist levels in the "A", the therapist interprets the meaning of these in her assessment. She feels that these items show progress.

A: Patient demonstrates improved w/c mobility from mod Ⓐ last Thursday to min Ⓐ today. Pt. also demonstrates ↑ AROM in all 5 digits and ↑ activity tolerance in wrist extension (x10 repetitions) from last Thursday (x5 repetitions).

This OTA basically plans to continue with the same program since she is seeing good progress.

A: Patient demonstrates improved w/c mobility from mod Ⓐ last Thursday to min Ⓐ today. Pt. also demonstrates ↑ AROM in all 5 digits and ↑ activity tolerance in wrist extension (x10 repetitions) from last Thursday (x5 repetitions). Pt. would benefit from further strengthening and AROM to reach the 4+ UE strength and ¾ AROM needed for independence in ADL tasks.

A program of routine exercises is not billable as skilled occupational therapy. Therefore, this OTA has shifted the responsibility for the exercise program to a restorative aide because the exercise program is now in place and the patient is able to do it correctly.

P: Continue Ⓑ UE exercises daily for 1 wk under supervision of a restorative aide to ↑ strength, activity tolerance, and AROM.

She plans to continue seeing the patient and to use the treatment sessions to accomplish the other goals that require the skill of an OTA. The goal she establishes is related to the sessions she will carry out based on the performance components that are being addressed by the restorative aide.

P: Continue skilled OT 3x wk for work on specific ADL of dressing, grooming, hygiene @ 1 hr./visit.

She ends the note with the short-term goal.

P: Continue Ⓑ UE exercises daily for 1 wk under supervision of a restorative aide to ↑ strength, activity tolerance, and AROM. Continue skilled OT 3x wk for work on specific ADLs of dressing, bathing, grooming @ 1 hr./visit. Pt. will be Ⓘ in ADL tasks by discharge in 2 weeks.

Worksheet 6-4

A Treatment Session Devoted to ADL Activities

S: Resident asked for help toileting. He responded to being addressed by name and indicated that it was time for his therapy. He was able to indicate the date and the time of day using a clock and calendar.

O: Resident seen in room to work on dressing and toileting activities. Resident required verbal, written, and tactile cues throughout the session to maintain balance. When sitting on edge of bed patient was dependent in donning underwear and coveralls over feet due to unstable balance. He required mod Ⓐ x2 sit → stand and to maintain static postural control. Mod Ⓐ required to complete donning of underwear and coveralls over hips and to place arms in armholes of coveralls while standing. After sitting, resident Ⓓ with zipping and fastening 2 snaps to fasten coveralls 2° fatigue. When performing toileting task, patient required max Ⓐ to transfer from w/c → standing pivot → toilet. Patient needed max Ⓐ x1 to maintain postural control to doff/don underwear and coveralls to knee level.

Write your own "A" and "P" section for the ADL note.

A:

P:

Helpful Hints

- Look at every sentence in the "S" and the "O" and decide what each might mean.
- For your "A," decide what problems, progress and rehab potential you see in this observation. What performance areas are impacted by performance components not WFL? What treatment do you think would benefit the patient?
- For your "P," consider what would you expect to see him able to do in the next week or two.

Chapter Seven

Goals and Interventions

In *Chapter Six: Writing the "P"—Plan*, you learned how to end the SOAP note with a short-term or long-term goal, identifying the specific treatment the patient will be receiving next in therapy. Now we will look more closely at the subject of writing good occupational therapy goals and developing intervention strategies from those goals. A clear understanding of these concepts will improve your documentation skills as well as enhance your ability to think and plan as an OTA.

Goals

The goals and objectives that are used in the documentation of occupational therapy services must be written in functional, measurable, observable, action-oriented terms. They must also be realistic for the patient, and achievable in a "reasonable" amount of time. For successful treatment, it is critical that you work on goals that are important to the patient. Occupational therapy goals must focus on functional gains. The component or biomechanical gains that underlie such progress are much less important to a third party payer than what the patient can actually do, even though the gains in performance components may be essential to achieving the functional outcome.

Long-Term Goals

Goals in a treatment plan are also called *long-term goals* (LTGs) or outcomes. They are formulated by the OT from the problem list that was compiled in collaboration with the patient during the initial assessment. These are usually discharge goals—what the OT hopes to see the patient accomplish by the time of discharge. For each problem that has been identified, there will be at least one LTG, and often more than one. An OTA will use these goals to develop specific treatments that will help the patient successfully reach these outcomes by the time occupational therapy services are discontinued. Goals are also used by an OTA when documenting the patient's progress. With each SOAP note that is written, an OTA records what the patient said, what the patient did, and what progress (or lack of progress) was made in relation to the goals that were identified in the initial assessment.

Short-Term Goals

Objectives are also called *short-term goals* (STGs). These are the daily or weekly goals that are met while progressing toward the discharge goals. In documentation of the patient's treatment, the OTA will provide a record of which of the objectives have been met, then write new STGs to meet the LTGs of the treatment plan. Again, the OTA will receive supervision from the OT in performing this function. The level of supervision will vary depending on the OTA's level of experience and demonstration of competency in this role (AOTA, 1993).

Writing Short-Term Goals or Objectives

The STGs are developed from the LTGs of the treatment plan. They are the "steps" that you will use to move the patient toward the established outcome. These objectives need to be measurable, observable, and client-oriented (Figure 7-1).

For example, if the LTG in the initial evaluation is:

> *In order to perform a job without injury, pt. will be able to move 35# objects needed for work from table to counter without ↑ in pain by 12/18/02.*

Then one of your STGs might be:

> *In order to perform tasks of job, pt. will be able to lift 10# objects needed for work without ↑ in pain by 12/5/02.*

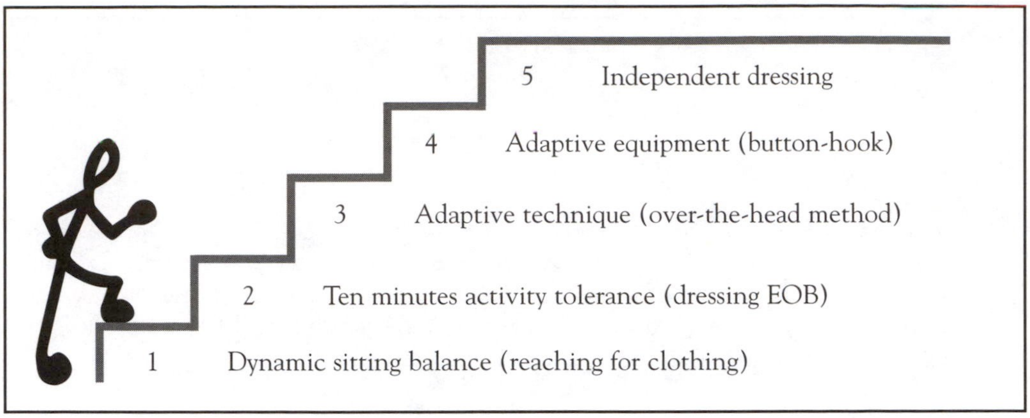

Figure 7-1. Steps to the ultimate LTG.

If the LTG is:

In order to return to independent living situation, pt. will transfer independently and safely bed ⇄ wheelchair standing pivot, and wearing an orthotic foot support within 2 weeks.

Then one of your STGs might be:

In order to be independent and safe in standing pivot transfers required for returning home, pt. will reach for bed or wheelchair before sitting with no verbal cues within 1 week.

The FEAST Method

In order to write goals and objectives in a way that can be measured, the elements to be included are very specific. The FEAST method is useful as you are learning to write (Table 7-1). The order may need to be changed slightly in order for your sentence to make sense. As long as all of the required elements are present, you can begin with any of the elements—the expectation, the conditions, the timeline, or the function. Now let's look at each category a little more closely.

F (Function)

This is the specific performance area to which this goal pertains, if it is not imbedded in the goal (i.e., "...in order to be able to dress self with minimum assist," or "in order to return to work as a carpenter," or "in order to be able to be bathed by his caretakers," or "in order to be able to write his name.")

For example:

In order to begin writing his name, the student will demonstrate ability to hold a crayon using tripod pinch by 3/19/02.

The function may go after the action if you prefer. For example:

The student will be able to hold a crayon using tripod pinch in order to write his name by 3/19/02.

Often the function is the same as the action.

The patient will perform a three step cooking process at wheelchair level by 3/16/02.

In this case the function (cooking) is inherent in the goal and does not need to be restated.

Function is the core of occupational therapy practice. It is the first thing you think of in writing goals, and should be the essential focus of the goal statement.

E (Expectation)

In writing treatment goals, the patient is the key player. You set the expectation:

The patient will...

A (Action)

Note: These are the patient's goals. The goal statement is not the place to tell what the therapist will do. That goes later, under intervention strategies.

An action verb is inserted here such as perform, demonstrate, identify, cook, don, comb, unfasten, or complete to describe the action or behavior the patient will accomplish. Describing the skill to be performed completes the statement. Usually the function is contained in the action statement, and does not need to be added.

Table 7-1

Goal Writing: FEAST Method

F—Function	For what functional gain?
E—Expectation	The patient will?
A—Action	Do what?
S—Specific conditions	Under what conditions?
T—Timeline	By when?

For example:

The patient will perform a three-step cooking process.

Statements using passive verbs do not provide observable actions or behaviors and are not used. For example, instead of using a passive verb, "patient will learn energy conservation techniques", use an action statement to communicate the action to be achieved; "patient will correctly demonstrate energy conservation techniques when dressing."

S (Specific Conditions)

This is the level of assistance expected and/or the conditions under which the patient is expected to be able to perform the desired action. For example: "...after set up"; "...3 out of 4 times"; "...by using a dressing stick"; "...at wheelchair level"; "...after skilled instruction."

The patient will perform a three-step cooking process at wheelchair level...

The conditions make your goal more specific. Usually it is helpful to put the condition after the skill rather than before it, but sometimes you may want to start with the condition. For example:

After skilled instruction the patient will be able to perform a three-step cooking process without cues.

Using the number of successful task completions in relation to attempts provides a goal that is measurable and specific. Percentages are more difficult to quantify and do not provide information on the number of trials that were necessary before success was achieved.

Patent will don and doff pants while maintaining total hip precautions without verbal cues 3/3 consecutive trials.

The following are some examples of goals in which the conditions have been italicized for emphasis. One of the most common mistakes in goal writing is omission of the conditions under which the activity is expected to be performed.

In order to dress himself with minimum assistance, pt. will button at least three buttons on his shirt **using a buttonhook** by 3/1/02.

In order to be able to begin dressing training by 11/30/02, pt. will maintain static sitting balance Ⓘ for 3 minutes **on side of bed.**

After initial prompt, pt. will greet 3 members of group by name.

After skilled instruction, pt. will demonstrate proper use of sock-aid to don socks Ⓘ safely while seated in w/c by end of 6th treatment session.

In order to don pants **completely over hips** pt. will demonstrate ability to transfer sit ↔ stand Ⓘ within 4 weeks.

Using the number of cues or the assist level as a part of the goal allows you to grade the activity and to show progress over time. For example, your LTG might be independence in the activity. Your STG might be mod Ⓐ this week, and min Ⓐ the following week in that same activity.

T (Timeline)

This is the time frame within which the goal is expected to be accomplished. For example: "...by discharge on 3/16/02" or "...by the end of the next treatment session," or "...within 2 weeks."

The patient will perform a three-step cooking process at wheelchair level without cues by 3/16/02.

Educational Goals

Therapists working in the public schools use a slightly different terminology. In education, goals for one school year are called "objectives." Educational goals are not measured by time, that is, by 5/7/02 or within 3 weeks. Since the IEP is rewritten annually, the time frame for educational goals is assumed to be annual. Children sometimes exhibit a new behavior inconsistently before it is really established. Therefore, measurement used for children is more likely to reflect whether or not the behavior is established. For example:

Kevin will hold pencil in a tripod grasp in 3/3 opportunities.

Johnny will demonstrate improved tolerance to tactile media as evidenced by self-initiation during art activities in 5/5 teacher reports.

Goals for children in the public schools must be set in terms of a behavior that is needed in the classroom. While you may be working on sensory integration as a treatment goal, such as maintaining prone extension posture over a therapy ball, it must be written in language that relates to performance in the classroom setting.

Bobby will maintain upright sitting posture during a 10-minute writing time without verbal reminders in 3/3 observations.

Do not use participation in treatment as a goal. For example:

Pt. will do 20 reps of shoulder ladder with 1# wt. in order to ↑ endurance to become more Ⓘ in ADLs.

In a goal such as this, specify the amount of ↑ endurance you hope or expect to see. For example:

Pt. will be able to participate in cooking task >5 minutes without rest breaks.

Examples of Well-Written Goal Statements

ADL Skills

- Pt. will be able to unfasten 3 out of 4 ½" buttons Ⓘ in less than 3 minutes within 2 weeks.
- Pt. will don socks with CGA using a sock-aid by 9/8/02.

Cognition

- Pt. will feed self a meal with correct use of adaptive equipment (lipped plate, rocker knife, and built-up angled utensils) after set-up with no more than 10 verbal cues by 9/11/02.
- Pt. will perform grooming with less than 3 verbal cues to redirect attention to task within 1 week.
- In order to grocery shop Ⓘ, pt. will locate proper aisle within 5 minutes of entering grocery store.

Edema

- Pt. will independently implement edema control techniques 5x during work shift by 4/9/02.
- In order to return to work as a typist, pt. will demonstrate 10% reduction in wrist circumference within 3 treatment sessions.

Activity Tolerance

- In order to complete morning ADL tasks, pt. will tolerate >10 minutes of activity with no more than one rest period by 10/19/02.
- In order to perform grooming tasks Ⓘ, pt. will tolerate >5 minutes of activity with Ⓛ hand with a reported pain level of <3/10 within 3 tx sessions.

Pain

- Pt. will comb hair Ⓘ s̄ c/o pain by the 5th treatment session.
- Pt. will complete grooming and hygiene activities with a reported pain level of <3/10 within 3 tx sessions.

Range of Motion

- Biomechanical goals are no longer used in many areas of clinical practice because of payment issues. Use functional goals instead, if possible.
- Pt. will demonstrate ↑ shoulder flexion PROM to 90° and abduction to 50° in order to don shirt with min Ⓐ in 2 weeks.
- In order to button shirt Ⓘ, pt. will demonstrate Ⓡ thumb MP flexion of no less than 50° within 2 weeks.

Return to Work

- In order to return to carpentry work, pt. will demonstrate Ⓡ UE grip strength >70# within 4 weeks.

Safety

- After skilled instruction, patient will demonstrate an ability to shower safely using adaptive equipment with mod Ⓐ within 2 weeks.
- In order to return to living unassisted, patient will demonstrate an ability to locate phone numbers of emergency services in the telephone directory Ⓘ after the 3rd treatment session.

Transfers/Mobility

- Within 4 weeks, pt. will perform a pivot transfer mod Ⓐ from bed to wheelchair in order to be Ⓘ in toileting.
- In order to return to living at home, pt. will be able to propel w/c up ramp and through all doors with min Ⓐ within 2 weeks.

Mental Health and Substance Abuse

- Consumer will Ⓘ prepare a TV dinner in the microwave within 1 week.
- Consumer will Ⓘ request a job application from a restaurant within 1 week.
- Consumer will take a shower without prompting at least 4x wk by 7/12/02.
- With mod verbal cues, consumer will ask roommate to smoke outside the building.
- Client will develop a plan for leisure time that does not include drinking by 4/8/02.

Worksheet 7-1

Evaluating Goal Statements

Which of the following goals has each of the necessary components to be useful in occupational therapy documentation? For each goal that you find to be incomplete or inaccurate in some way, indicate what is lacking.

1. By the time of discharge in 2 weeks, patient will be able to dress himself with min Ⓐ for balance using a sock aid and reacher while sitting in a wheelchair.

   __ This goal has all the necessary components to be useful.
   __ This goal lacks ____.

2. Patient will tolerate 10 minutes of treatment daily.

   __ This goal has all the necessary components to be useful.
   __ This goal lacks ____.

3. Patient will demonstrate increased coping skills in order to live at home with her granddaughter within 2 weeks.

   __ This goal has all the necessary components to be useful.
   __ This goal lacks ____.

4. Patient will demonstrate 15 minutes of activity tolerance without rest breaks using Ⓑ UE in order to complete ADL tasks before breakfast each morning.

   __ This goal has all the necessary components to be useful.
   __ This goal lacks ____.

5. In order to be able to toilet self Ⓘ after discharge, patient will demonstrate ability to perform a sliding board transfer w/c ↔ mat within the next week.

   __ This goal has all the necessary components to be useful.
   __ This goal lacks ____.

6. OT will teach lower body dressing using a reacher, dressing stick, and sock aid within 3 tx sessions.

   __ This goal has all the necessary components to be useful.
   __ This goal lacks ____.

7. In order to return to living independently, pt. will demonstrate ability to balance his checkbook.

   __ This goal has all the necessary components to be useful.
   __ This goal lacks ____.

Worksheet 7-2

Writing Realistic, Functional, and Measurable Goals

Rewrite the following goals to be measurable, functional, time-limited, and action-oriented, and specify the conditions under which the action is to occur. Without knowing more details about the patient, it is impossible to know what the goal would be. For purposes of this exercise, just imagine a patient and decide what the goal might be, then practice wording it correctly.

Increase Attention Span

F (if not included in action below)________________________________
(For what functional gain)

E ____
(Expectation—the patient will)

A ____
(Action)

S ____
(Specific Conditions)

T ____
(Timeline—by when?)

Teach the Patient to Follow Directions

F (if not included in action below)________________________________

E ____

A ____

S ____

T ____

Pt. to Dress Upper Body

F (if not included in action below)________________________________

E ____

A ____

S ____

T ____

Increase Endurance

F (if not included in action below)____________________

E ____________________

A ____________________

S ____________________

T ____________________

Improve Money Management Skills

F (if not included in action below)____________________

E ____________________

A ____________________

S ____________________

T ____________________

Decrease Depression

F (if not included in action below)____________________

E ____________________

A ____________________

S ____________________

T ____________________

The Relationship of Goals to Interventions

Interventions

An intervention is a plan of action taken to achieve the stated goals and objectives that have been developed in the course of occupational therapy treatment. The OT is responsible for developing an intervention plan and treatment goals in the initial evaluation. In some settings, this initial evaluation will include the problem list along with LTGs, but not STGs or interventions. Under the supervision of an OT, an OTA can put this plan into practice, using "specific purposeful activities or therapeutic methods that are meaningful to the client and are effective methods for enhancing occupational performance" (AOTA, 1998, p. 868). In doing this, the OTA should also be able to develop and write STGs from the LTGs provided in the initial evaluation. As treatment proceeds, changes to the plan may be necessary because of changes in the patient's status or unexpected responses to the treatment thus far. An OTA may help identify the need for changes and contribute to the intervention modification under the OT's supervision (AOTA, 1998).

Here is an example of a treatment plan, which would be included as a part of the initial evaluation.

Goal	Interventions
STG: Pt. will be able to complete basic ADL tasks while standing for 5-minute increments and taking rest breaks as needed by discharge date 3/20/02.	• Set up task to make coffee while standing at counter in the ADL kitchen. • Instruct pt. to stand at the bathroom sink to wash hands after toileting. • Instruct pt. to stand in a standing table to play a game. • Instruct pt. to stand to arrange clothing while dressing in the AM. • Instruct pt. to stand to look out window to watch birds eat the food she has put out.
STG: Pt. will be able to manage her financial affairs Ⓘ in order to live alone after anticipated discharge on 3/20/02. Teach basic math skills (add, subtract, multiply, divide).	• Role play to make change correctly. • Set up task for writing checks to pay fabricated bills. • Teach comparison shopping using a catalog. • Set up task of writing out a budget. • Set up task of balancing a checkbook. • Set up experience for deciding whether a given amount of money will be enough for living expenses once a set of fabricated bills has been paid.

As you can see, goals and interventions are not identical. **Goals** are stated from the patient's point of view, in terms of what the patient will accomplish. **Interventions** are stated from the therapist's point of view, in terms of what the therapist will do to help the patient meet the stated goals. Using this description, the differences are clear. However, sometimes an inexperienced OTA may have difficulty in distinguishing between goals and interventions, which may result in documentation that does not communicate the occupational therapy process in a clear and concise manner.

- A **goal** must be behavioral and measurable to be useful. For example, "Pt. will Ⓘ propel w/c 10 ft. to bathroom within 3 days" is a goal.
- An **intervention** is written so that another person will clearly understand what activities are to be used with the patient. "Instruct patient in how to use feet to propel w/c", is an intervention. There is no specific formula for wording an intervention as there is for a goal. Interventions need to be clearly understandable to the person who is expected to carry them out.

Which of the following statements are goals and which are interventions?

1. Pt. will be able to dress lower body Ⓘ sitting EOB by 7/9/02.
2. Use Brunnstrom exercises to ↑ UE PROM.
3. Pt. to propel w/c to gift shop.

The first statement is a goal. The second is an intervention. The third statement is not really specific enough to be either one, but with some modification could become either a goal or an intervention. If it were written "Pt. will be able to propel w/c to gift shop Ⓘ without running into wall within 3 days" it would be a goal. If it were written "Instruct patient to turn head to Ⓛ when propelling w/c to avoid running into walls" it would be an intervention.

Earlier in this chapter you learned about writing goals that are written in functional, measurable, observable, action-oriented terms. In the following section, you will be generating intervention strategies to help the patient meet those clearly-written goals. It is beyond the scope of this book to teach intervention, and these exercises are not meant to be comprehensive. The following exercises are designed to help you learn the differences between goals and interventions, and begin learning how to brainstorm in creating intervention strategies for those occasions that you have to "think on your feet " due to some unexpected event.

Worksheet 7-3

Mrs. Murphy's Wheelchair Mobility

Mrs. Murphy is an 84-year-old woman who has had a Ⓛ total hip replacement. She is not very good at problem-solving, and she will probably be going to a nursing home when she is discharged. Her wheelchair is a little large for her, and she has trouble propelling it. She has decreased strength, and needs verbal cues to avoid running into things. You will be picking up this patient tomorrow. The OT treated her last week and wrote this note. You will be providing her therapy for the remainder of her treatments. Use this note to answer the questions about goals and interventions that follow:

S: Pt. reported pain in Ⓛ hip and feeling tired.

O: Pt. was seen in room to address issues of functional mobility and activity tolerance needed to complete self-care tasks.

Functional mobility:

Patient required max Ⓐ supine → sit and EOB → w/c using a pivot transfer. To accommodate Ⓑ knee flexion contractures, pt. was repositioned in her w/c by using pillows behind her back, which allowed her to reach the floor more easily. Pt. required min Ⓐ to propel w/c due to problems straightening front casters prior to starting and after turning. Pt. demonstrated ability to propel w/c ~10 feet, turn w/c, and go through doorways, all with min Ⓐ to maneuver w/c around room for basic ADL tasks and for participating in activities at her residential care facility.

Activity tolerance: Pt. able to tolerate 15 minutes of activity starting from transferring from bed → w/c to propelling w/c in and out of room necessary for completion of self-care and leisure tasks.

A: Pain in Ⓛ hip and ↓ strength limit patient's ability to propel w/c independently. Bilateral knee flexion contractures interfere with patient's ability to transfer bed → w/c and supine → sit unassisted. Decreased functional mobility impairs patient's ability to complete basic self-care tasks, particularly lower body dressing Ⓘ. Good rehab potential is shown by patient's ability to propel chair with min Ⓐ to follow 1-step instructions and initiate activity. Pt. would benefit from continued training in functional mobility, education in compensatory techniques, and a w/c consult to get pt. a w/c that meets her needs.

P: Patient to be seen daily for the next week to address functional mobility and basic ADL tasks from w/c. OT will evaluate pt's w/c needs and contact vendor for new w/c if warranted. Pt. will be Ⓘ in w/c mobility by estimated d/c in 1 week.

Julia Patton, OTR

What is the goal for this patient?

What interventions might you use to help this patient become stronger and learn to propel her wheelchair more successfully?

Worksheet 7-4

Interrupted Interventions

Rehab Center Setting

Allen Jones is a 60-year-old male who has had a left CVA. He is getting some return in his involved right (dominant) upper extremity, and has some gross grasp, although fine motor tasks are still difficult. He has limited AROM and strength in the right shoulder. He is working on dressing in occupational therapy. This morning it was your plan to work on compensatory dressing techniques and correct use of adaptive equipment, but when you arrived in his room at 8:00 am, you found he had already been dressed by the nursing staff and was sitting in his wheelchair. What might you do instead of helping him get dressed that would make good use of his treatment time and would work toward his goals of increasing independence in dressing?

1.

2

3.

4.

Mental Health Setting

Bill is a divorced 57-year-old male who was admitted to the psych unit yesterday for depression and alcohol use. Initial evaluation shows that he has low self-esteem, no friends, and no reported interests other than drinking. Goals established by the OT include improving his self-esteem as well as developing social and leisure skills that do not involve alcohol use. This afternoon he was scheduled to play volleyball in recreation, but yesterday he fractured his collar bone, and will not be able to participate in active games until it is healed. He has been sent to occupational therapy in place of the volleyball game. What might you do to work on his goals of self-esteem and social and leisure skills?

1.

2.

Chapter Eight

Documenting Different Stages of Treatment

As we discussed in *Chapter One: Documenting the Treatment Process in Occupational Therapy*, different stages of the treatment process require occupational therapists to write different kinds of notes. Very early in the process, an **intake note** may be written by an OT acknowledging the referral and stating a plan to evaluate. Next, an **initial evaluation report** is written, reporting the findings from the OT's evaluation of the patient and detailing a problem list. From this comes the **treatment plan**, which is developed by the OT and is technically a part of the initial evaluation report. After the initial evaluation is written, treatment begins and notes are written that provide regular documentation of the patient's progress in achieving the goals that were established. Facilities vary in the type and frequency of documentation required. Some settings, such as home health and outpatient clinics, require a **treatment note** for each visit. Others, such as a mental health clinic, require **progress notes** at least weekly, and more often if changes in status indicate. Long-term care residential facilities usually require a progress note every 30 days, and more frequently for new referrals. The requirements for type and frequency of notes are usually a function of the accrediting agency and the payment source. Sometimes an OT is required to write a **reassessment note** at regular intervals. As treatment ends, most facilities require a **discharge report**. Again, as stated in Chapter One, specific guidelines for the particular roles of the OT and OTA in documentation of services are dependent upon the particular facility, accrediting or state agency and third party payers that are involved in the delivery of the occupational therapy services (Backhaus and Sladyk, 2001).

In actual practice, you will find that treatment, progress, and reassessment notes may have some overlap. For example, in outpatient settings the treatment notes often include the client's progress. Treatment notes in other settings where patients may change quickly, such as acute care, may also read much like progress notes. In some ways, progress notes reassess the patient and may sound much like reassessment notes. There are some guidelines for each kind of note, however, and in this chapter we will examine the requirements for documentation at each stage of patient care.

In *Elements of Clinical Documentation* (Revision) (Thomson & Foto, 1995) criteria for five kinds of notes are described—the initial evaluation report (including the treatment plan), treatment notes (also called visit or contact notes), progress reports, reevaluation reports, and discharge or discontinuation reports. In the following exercises we will compare some samples of each of these notes and see how well they stand up to the principles we have learned from previous chapters.

Initial Evaluation Reports

While OTAs will not be performing and writing initial evaluations, they will need to have a working knowledge of the process and content of these notes. These evaluations provide the information that is critical to OTAs as they begin therapy, containing patient data such as current diagnosis, treatment diagnosis, date of onset, and precautions or contraindications. The problems and goals noted in the "A" and "P" sections of the initial evaluation will form the foundation of the treatment plan. From these problems and goals, intervention strategies are chosen that will move the patient toward the goals that were established by the OT in the initial evaluation.

After a referral form is received on a patient, the OT begins the evaluation process to determine what that patient needs from occupational therapy. First, data is collected from the patient, the family, the chart, and any other pertinent sources. Then standardized tests or survey instruments are selected and administered to help determine exactly what needs to be done. From the initial evaluation reports, the OT identifies and prioritizes the performance areas and performance components that are to be treated, and develops a treatment plan. The three elements making up the initial evaluation report as listed in the *Elements of Clinical Documentation* (Revision) (Thomson & Foto, 1995) are as follows:

1. The identifying data and background information.
2. The tests performed and clinical observations, followed by an assessment of the results.
3. The treatment plan.

Most facilities provide a form for an initial evaluation report, and the evaluation results are recorded on the form, along with comments and observations. Some facilities use the same form for discharge notes so that the evaluation material does not have to be rewritten. The evaluation discharge form from Capital Region Medical Center in Jefferson City, MO is included so you can see what might be included on a good facility form (Figures 8-1a and b). You will notice that it has the performance area evaluations first, followed by performance components, with room for individualization.

If an OT writes an initial evaluation as a SOAP note, the information may be organized in the following manner:

S: The interview material

Depending upon the patient's cognitive abilities, the OT might ask about functioning in all performance areas (ADL, work, and leisure) to determine which are important to the patient and payer, and which areas are not WFL in the opinion of the patient. The interview will also reveal how the patient feels about the problem areas. There may be symbolic losses to consider, as well as physical losses. If a young child is being evaluated, or a patient whose cognitive function is not adequate to provide this information, this portion of the note will need to be supplemented with information provided by the primary caregivers.

O: The test results and clinical observations

This section includes the results of any survey instruments or standardized tests that have been performed (such as an ADL evaluation, developmental testing, goniometric evaluation, etc.) along with the clinical observations of the OT during the evaluation process. The tests selected by the OT will depend entirely on the kind of patient, the presenting problem, and the situation at the time of the evaluation. Different evaluation tests are used in a long-term care facility, for example, than would be used in a public school setting or in a mental health center.

A: The professional assessment of the data presented in the "S" and the "O"

In this section of the initial evaluation note, the OT will present his/her interpretation of the impact of the "O" data on the patient's occupational performance. Performance areas and the performance components that are not WFL are found here, including the type and severity of the limitations and the occupational performance deficits caused by these impairments. The OT will also set the priorities in this portion of the evaluation, determine rehab potential and justify the need for skilled OT.

Some facilities ask for a problem list in this section of the note. In a facility that uses a POMR, the problem list will be a separate document. In some settings (such as mental health centers and public school) the problem list is multidisciplinary. The problem list must be included somewhere in the OT record, as it will be the basis for formulating a treatment plan, with each problem being expanded to include long- and short-term goals and interventions to address the stated problem. Some facilities put the long- and short-term goals in the "A" section of the note, although most put them under the "P."

P: The frequency and duration of planned treatment and the long- and short-term goals

If the long- and short-term goals for the patient have not already been noted, they would be included at this point under the "P." This is the part of the note where the OT will set priorities. Safety, for example, is often a top priority. Reduction of pain is often another high priority item. Some kinds of performance components are prerequisites for the development of other skills. For example, sitting balance is a prerequisite for any task that must be done while sitting. Function is critical to the plan. OTs and OTAs are reimbursed for increasing occupational performance, and this must be reflected in the plan.

Discharge planning also begins with the initial evaluation. From the inception of care, the OT team is planning toward the probable discharge situation. This may change over the course of the patient's time in occupational therapy, but it is always a consideration.

CAPITAL REGION MEDICAL CENTER
OCCUPATIONAL THERAPY
❑ INITIAL EVALUATION ❑ DISCHARGE SUMMARY

DIAGNOSIS ______________________ ONSET: ______________

____

MED. HX: ______________________________________

______________________________ CODE STATUS: ______

RELEVANT SURG. PROC.: __________________________

REFERRAL DATE: ______________ DATE: ______________

REFERRING PHYSICIAN: ___________ MEDICARE #: ___________

ACTIVITIES OF DAILY LIVING REHAB POTENTIAL: ______________________

DRESSING Put on & remove the following	INDEP	SBA	MIN. ASSIST	MOD. ASSIST	MAX. ASSIST	ADAPT. EQUIP.	COMMENTS/ADAPTIVE EQUIPMENT ISSUED
front opening shirt							
pull on shirt							
underwear							
bra							
pants/slacks							
socks/hose							
shoes							
manage fasteners							
braces/splints/prosthesis							
GROOMING/HYGIENE							
sponge bath							
tub/shower bath							
shave							
comb hair							
brushing teeth							
opens jars/bottles							
make-up							
EATING							
drink from cup/glass							
feeds self							
cuts meat							

ROM				UPPER EXTREMITY ROM & STRENGTH		STRENGTH	
ACTIVE LEFT	PASSIVE LEFT	ACTIVE RIGHT	PASSIVE RIGHT			L	R
				SHOULDER:	Elevation		
					Flexion		
					Abduction		
					Horizontal Abduction		
					Horizontal Adduction		
					Internal Rotation		
					External Rotation		
				ELBOW:	Flexion		
					Extension		
					Supination		
					Pronation		
				WRIST:	Flexion		
				Shoulder Subluxation	L	R	
				UE Edema	L	R	
				Pain	L	R	

PERTINENT FINDINGS

Wears glasses_______ Dentures_______ Hearing_______

MUSCLE TONE/UPPER EXTREMITIES

Hypotonic_______ Normal_______ Hypertonic_______

Comments______________________

UPPER EXTREMITY SENSATION

SENSATION	Intact	Impaired	Absent
Light touch			
Sharp/Dull			
Temperature			
Proprioception			
Stereognosis			

COORDINATION/UPPER EXTREMITIES

Tremors_______ Apraxia_______ Ataxic_______

	Impaired	WNL
Gross Motor		
Fine Motor		

9 Hole Peg Test	L	R
Grip Strength	L	R
Lateral Pinch	L	R
Tripod Pinch	L	R
Hand Dominance	L	R

SURVIVAL SKILLS	Indep.	Min. Assist	Mod. Assist	Max. Assist
Phone Book Usage				
Money Mngmt.				
Situational Problem Solving				
Homemaking				

ORIENTED TO:

Person_______ Place_______
Time: Month_____ Day_____ Year_____
Situation_______

COMMUNICATION/COGNITION

	YES	NO
Verbal		
Understandable		
Appropriate		
Perseveration		
Follows Simple Commands		
Reads		
Writes		

PERCEPTION

A. R/L Neglect_______

	Impaired	WNL
B. Body Schema		
C. Discrimination		
Shape		
Size		
Color		
D. Visual Perception		

Overall Endurance WFL_______
Fair_______
Poor_______

2,605,003 (9/99) INIT. EVAL/DISCHG. SUM. (FRONT)

Figure 8-1a. Occupational therapy initial evaluation and discharge summary form (page 1). (Courtesy of Capital Region Medical Center, Jefferson City, MO.)

HOME SITUATION: ____________________

LIVING ARRANGEMENTS: (PT ADDRESS) ____________________

HOME TYPE: ____________________

PRIOR FUNCTIONAL INDEP.: ____________________

____

____

LEISURE INTERESTS: ____________________

ADAPTIVE EQUIP.: ____________________

COMMENTS: ____________________

____

____

____

PATIENT / FAMILY GOALS: ____________________

❑ INITIAL ASSESSMENT (PROBLEMS / STRENGTHS) ❑ DISCHARGE STATUS OF SHORT / LONG TERM GOALS

____

____

____

____

____

PLAN: ____________________

SHORT-TERM GOALS - ESTIMATED TIME TO ACHIEVE: ____________________

____

____

____

____

____

❑ LONG-TERM GOALS - ESTIMATED TIME TO ACHIEVE: ❑ RECOMMENDATIONS:

____

____

____

____

____

❑ Yes ❑ No **Patient has participated in evaluation process and agrees with treatment plan as stated above.**

Therapist ____________________ Date____________

I have reviewed and agree with the treatment plan as stated above.

Physician Signature ____________________ Date____________

2,605,003 (9/99) OT INITIAL EVALUATION/DISCHARGE SUMMARY (BACK)

Figure 8-1b. Occupational therapy initial evaluation and discharge summary form (page 2). (Courtesy of Capital Region Medical Center, Jefferson City, MO.)

Read the following initial evaluation report and treatment plan. Using the checklist in Worksheet 8-1, identify the data listed to assess your ability to find the pertinent information contained within this evaluation.

HOSPITAL AND REHABILITATION CENTER OCCUPATIONAL THERAPY

Initial Evaluation Report

Name: Agnes H. Age: 68 **Sex:** F **Physician:** T. Quay, MD **Date of Onset:** 2/1/01
Date of Admission: 2/2/01 **Date of Evaluation:** 2/3/01 **Time:** 10 am
History: Pt. referred by Dr. Quay for evaluation and treatment. She was admitted after a fall resulting in confusion and left-sided weakness. Prior to admission she was living alone and was Ⓘ in all activities of daily living.
Primary Diagnosis: Ⓡ CVA r/o OBS **Secondary Diagnosis:** diabetes

S: Pt. stated, "I'm doing this so I can go home."

O: Pt. seen at bedside for mini-mental status exam, manual muscle test, AROM, strength, and functional mobility. Pt. also seen in shower room for toileting, dressing/undressing, and showering.

Bathing: Upper body: min Ⓐ Lower body: min Ⓐ except max Ⓐ for perineal area and feet.

Dressing: Seated in chair with arms, min Ⓐ with verbal cues except for mod Ⓐ to initiate donning bra, and max Ⓐ for shoes and socks. Verbal cues needed for sequencing and environment orientation.

Toileting: Verbal cues to flush, min Ⓐ to obtain tissue and manage clothing.

Transfers: CGA with verbal cues for safety/proper arm placement sit to stand; min Ⓐ from low surfaces.

Bed Mobility: Rolls & supine ⇄ sit SBA.

Standing Balance: static: CGA.

Activity Tolerance: fair (3, 1-5 scale) 10 minutes max tolerance to any activity with physical/mental challenges.

Motor Planning/Perception: WFLs.

Cognition: Score of 17/30 on MME. Sequencing problems during dressing tasks noted. Pt. could not attach bra in back and required verbal cues to attach in front.

UE AROM: WFLs for all Ⓑ UE movements except: Ⓛ shoulder: abd 0-30°, int/ext rotation 0-45°.

UE Strength: Grip: Ⓡ 42 lbs. Ⓛ 21 lbs. Pinch: Ⓡ palmar 14#; Ⓡ lateral 15#; Ⓛ palmar 6 #; Ⓛ lateral 8#.

Manual Muscle Test: All movements 4/5 except Ⓛ elbow ext. 3/5, thumb opposition and abduction 3+.

Sensation: Ⓛ UE: Light touch, pain, temperature intact; Stereognosis 3/5 Ⓡ UE all intact.

A: Pt. problem-solved poorly while undressing, (trying to doff pants prior to doffing shoes/socks) and during dressing to initiate an alternative way to don bra. Pt. displayed Ⓛ UE ↓ AROM, ↓ strength, slow cognition and sequencing and problem-solving strategies. Pt. has ↓ short-term memory, which is a safety concern. Due to ↓ cognition pt. requires verbal cues to initiate some ADL tasks. Pt. would benefit from environmental cues to orient her to environment, problem-solving, and sequencing activities, and activities to ↑ AROM and strength in the Ⓛ UE. Rehab potential is good for modified Ⓘ in ADL activities.

P: Pt. will be seen for 45-minute sessions 5 x/wk for 2 wks for sequencing during ADL tasks, problem-solving strategies, activities to ↑ activity tolerance, AROM and strength in Ⓛ UE. Put calendar in pt.'s room to increase orientation to month, day, and season. Pt. will be able to dress with SBA and <3 verbal cues after set-up within 2 weeks.

Treatment Plan

Problem #1: Pt. needs min to max physical assist and verbal cues to dress self due to ↓ AROM, activity tolerance, and ability to sequence the task.

LTG: Pt. will be able to dress with SBA and <3 verbal cues after set-up within 2 weeks.

Objective	Interventions
STG: Pt. will don bra Ⓘ using adapted technique within 1 week.	• Teach adaptive techniques. • Post picture of how to don bra correctly using adapted technique. • Reinforce correct responses. • Teach coordination exercises.
STG: Pt. will don shoes and socks Ⓘ using adapted technique and a long shoehorn within 1½ weeks.	• Provide long shoehorn and instruct pt. in correct use. • Instruct in adapted techniques for donning shoes and socks. • Post picture of adapted technique and long shoehorn being used to don shoes. • Instruct in using affected side as a functional assist in dressing. • Expand exercise program to include AROM and strength.
STG: Pt. will sequence dressing tasks correctly 3/3 tries within 2 weeks.	• Verbalize steps before beginning to dress. • Verbalize steps while dressing. • Post list of steps for pt. to follow. • Take rest breaks as needed for activity tolerance.

Problem #2: Pt.'s lack of orientation to environment and inability to problem-solve cause safety concerns with ADL and home management.

LTG: Pt. will correctly use calendar, schedule, clock, and emergency information posted on wall within 2 weeks.

Objective	Interventions
STG: Pt. will correctly identify time, date, and situation when asked within 1 week.	• Post calendar, schedule, and emergency information near clock in pt.'s room. • Instruct nursing staff and other therapy staff to ask pt. date, time, and situation several times daily and to reinforce correct responses.
STG: Pt. will be able to follow a daily schedule with < 2 verbal cues/day within 1½ weeks.	• Post daily schedule on wall near clock. • Cue pt. to look at schedule to determine what she should be doing at any given time.
STG: Pt. will correctly problem-solve responses to emergency situations in 9/10 tries within 2 weeks.	• Provide situations for patient to problem-solve, progressing from easy to more complex. • Provide telephone directory or other props as needed for problem-solving.

Tara Grantham, OTR

Worksheet 8-1

Initial Evaluation Report

In each section on the right side of the checklist, make a note of the information found in the preceding initial evaluation.

Background Data

Is the basic demographic data (name, age, sex, date of onset, date of admission, date of referral) present? Note any not present.	
Who referred the patient to OT and what services were requested?	
Is the patient's medical history and prior level of function included?	
What secondary problems, pre-existing conditions, contraindications, or precautions exist that will impact therapy?	
What life stage or environmental factors will impact treatment?	
Is the current level of function assessed?	
What do the consumer and her family expect or want from treatment?	

Adapted from Elements of Clinical Documentation *(Revision) (Thomson & Foto, 1995)*

Results of the Assessment

What tests were used? Were there any deviations from the standard procedures?	
What other information or observations were collected besides those from the tests?	
Are the impairments and their severity identified?	
Are the functional limitations stated in objective and measurable terms?	
What is the rehab potential for this patient?	

Adapted from Elements of Clinical Documentation *(Revision) (Thomson & Foto, 1995)*

Treatment Plan

List one of the functional, measurable long-term goals for this patient.	
Are the long-term goals reasonable in relation to the consumer's current status, rehabilitation status, and prior level of functioning?	
What documentation is there that the patient and family agree with the goals?	
Do the short-term goals (objectives) relate to the long-term goals?	
List one of the short-term goals for problem #2.	
Are the interventions that have been selected appropriate to meet the goals?	
What assistive devices are to be used?	
What are the number, frequency, and duration of treatment sessions planned?	
Are there any recommendations or referrals?	

Adapted from Elements of Clinical Documentation *(Revision) (Thomson & Foto, 1995)*

Progress Notes

Progress notes are written on a regularly scheduled basis (usually weekly or monthly) with the time frame determined by the facility. The facility is guided by the accrediting agencies and primary payers in setting the time intervals for these notes. The requirements for a progress note specify that the treatment interventions be noted, along with the consumer's response to them. There should be an explanation of goals that are modified, changed or continued, along with any changes in expected time frames. The effectiveness of treatment, including any adaptive devices, should be noted. Any conferences with others should be documented, any home programs should be attached, and any instruction given to caregivers should be noted, along with future plans (Thomson & Foto, 1995).

For example, the patient who was evaluated in the previous initial evaluation report was to begin receiving skilled occupational therapy 5 times a week for 2 weeks. The rehabilitation center where she is a patient requires weekly progress notes, so the OTA who provides her treatment for this first week may write a note like this:

S: Pt. states she likes having the calendar and activity schedule on her wall because "now I can tell what day it is." Nursing and other therapy staff report pt. has correctly identified date and time 4/5 times.

O: Pt. has been seen in her room 5x for ADL retraining, cognitive activities and therapeutic exercise to Ⓛ UE. Pt. initiates donning bra by hooking in front with 1-2 verbal cues to refer to illustration of the technique posted on her wall for correct sequencing. She dons shoes using long-handled shoehorn with min Ⓐ to insert horn into shoe. She requires mod Ⓐ to don/doff socks using Ⓛ side as a functional assist. She performs 15 minutes of self-care activities before requiring a rest break. Pt. refers to calendar and daily schedule posted on her wall and answers correctly 4/5 times when she is asked by staff and family for day or activity time, but she continues to give inappropriate responses to questions concerning emergency situations (such as inability to identify pathway to safety in case of fire). Therapeutic exercise Ⓛ UE includes using therapy putty to increase grasp and pinch strength with improvement as noted: Ⓛ grasp 25#; Ⓛ palmar pinch 10#, Ⓛ lateral pinch 12#.

A: Pt. has shown increased independence in dressing using adaptive equipment and techniques as instructed, along with posted illustrations of these techniques in her room. ↑ UE strength has ↑ function as demonstrated by her ability to hook her bra and manipulate the shoehorn. Orientation to her environment has improved with use of calendars, schedules, and reinforcement by staff, but her inability to problem-solve independently may pose safety concerns for independent living after discharge from this facility. Pt. would benefit from continued instruction and training in ADL and cognitive activities to ↑ her Ⓘ and safety $\bar{p}$ D/C.

P: Continue skilled OT 5x/week for 1 week for ADL retraining, problem-solving strategies and activities to ↑ strength and AROM in Ⓛ UE. Develop a home exercise program and give written and verbal instructions to pt. and daughter. Provide situations for patient to problem-solve, such as using telephone to call daughter to summon medical assistance, and finding pathway to safety in facility by anticipated D/C in 1 wk. Pt will be oriented to environment using calendar, clock, and schedule in room and will perform dressing activities SBA with 1-2 verbal cues after set-up in 1 wk.

Worksheet 8-2

Progress Notes

Using the following checklist, determine whether the preceding note meets the standards for progress notes.

Criteria	Compliance
What treatment interventions were used?	
What changes have occurred in this consumer?	
What goals have been continued, what goals have been changed, and what goals have been discontinued?	
Have there been any changes in the time frames for reaching goals?	
If any assistive devices are being used, how effective are these?	
What contact or conferences have there been with others?	
Is there a specific plan for the future?	

Adapted from Elements of Clinical Documentation *(Revision) (Thomson & Foto, 1995)*

Treatment Notes

Contact, visit, or treatment notes are used to document each visit or each individual occupational therapy session. In some situations, such as home health, contact notes are required in the medical record each time a patient is seen. In other cases, such as mental health, the therapist keeps attendance records and informal contact notes, which are then summarized into a progress note.

Contact notes should contain documentation of the attendance and participation of the consumer in therapy. If the consumer did not attend as scheduled, there should be a note of the reason therapy did not occur. The interventions used in therapy should be noted, along with the consumer's response. If any assistive or adaptive devices were used, these should be noted, along with their effectiveness. It is possible that some items will not apply in all situations. For example, in a mental health setting there may not be any assistive or adaptive equipment used.

Read the following treatment note and use Worksheet 8-3 to determine how well it meets the standards.

Hospital and Rehabilitation Center Acute Care Unit

Occupational Therapy Contact Note

Date: 4/14/00 Time: 8:30 AM

S: Pt. reports, "I feel fair today. I had a long night."

O: Pt. seen bedside in ICU for instruction in ADL tasks and AROM in Ⓡ UE. Pt. nodded his head when asked if ready to sit up; required mod Ⓐ supine → sit. Upon sitting O_2 saturation dropped to ~85%. Grooming, dressing, and UE AROM activities not completed 2° low O_2 levels. Pt. given min Ⓐ to return to supine. After ~2 minutes O_2 levels returned to ~95%. Pt. washed face p̄ set-up in supine and nodded when asked if that felt good.

A: Pt. able to tolerate a little more activity today than yesterday when he did not have tolerance for supine → sit. Pt. also appears more motivated to attempt therapy session. Activity tolerance still limited due to O_2 saturation levels upon exertion. Pt. would benefit from instruction in energy conservation as well as correct positioning to ↓ exertion ↑ activity tolerance for ADL tasks.

P: Continue skilled OT qid to ↑ activity tolerance and Ⓘ in ADL tasks for 5 days or until D/C. Pt. will complete grooming EOB c̄ rest breaks as needed within 2 treatment sessions.

Worksheet 8-3

Contact, Visit, or Treatment Notes

Using the following checklist, determine whether the note on the preceding page meets the standards for treatment notes.

Criteria	Compliance
What evidence is there of the patient's participation in OT treatment?	
What activities, techniques, or modalities were used in this treatment session?	
If any assistive or adaptive devices were used, is there documentation of whether these were fabricated, sold, or rented, their effectiveness, and what the instructions were for their use?	
How did this patient (consumer) respond to the treatment provided?	

Adapted from Elements of Clinical Documentation *(Revision) (Thomson & Foto, 1995)*

Reevaluation Reports

In some settings, patients must be reevaluated monthly or quarterly. This type of note is the responsibility of the OT, but an OTA may contribute to the reevaluation process (AOTA, 1998). The reevaluation report is a cross between a progress note and a discharge summary. The tests that were given initially are readministered and the results are compared with the results of the previous tests to determine the effectiveness of the treatment being provided. The goals and plans are revised at this time and new timelines are projected.

Read the reevaluation report that follows and use Worksheet 8-4 to determine how well it meets the AOTA criteria. In addition, see whether this note meets the other standards for a good OT note that you have been taught in the previous chapters of this manual.

Hospital and Rehabilitation Center Reevaluation Report

S: Pt. initially reported "numbness and tingling in fingers." During last tx session pt. reported his "Ⓛ hand feels much stronger now."

O: Pt. admitted to hospital on 1/26/02 for treatment of Ⓛ UE following closed head injury resulting from MVA. OT initial evaluation on 1/27/02. Reassessment on 2/5/02. ADL assessment attached.

Ⓡ UE: WNL

Ⓛ UE:

Date	1/26	2/5
Shoulder Flexion	F	F+
Shoulder Extension	F	G
Shoulder Abd	F	F+
Shoulder Add	F	N
Internal/External Rotation	F+	G
Horizontal Abd/Add	F	G
Elbow Flexion/Extension	F-	F+
Pronation	F-	F+
Supination	F-	G-
Wrist Flexion	F-	G-
Wrist Extension	F	G
Ⓛ Grip	30/30/25	40/40/35
Ⓛ Lateral Pinch	8/8/7	10/11/10
Ⓛ Palmar Pinch	6.5/6.5/7.5	8/7/8

Pt. has been seen b.i.d. to work on strengthening the Ⓛ UE using theraband, hand-held wt. exercises, and therapy putty to increase independence in both basic and instrumental ADLs. Pt. has also worked on improving standing balance and has been instructed in bathroom safety (as related to tub transfers and equipment needs), but has not yet demonstrated proficiency in this area due to ↓ balance and activity tolerance.

A: Pt. Ⓛ muscle strength, grip strength, and prehension patterns have all improved. Pt. now able to continue exercise program under supervision of rehab aide.

Goals #1 and #2 are met.

Goal #3 (balance) not yet met.

Goal #4 (min Ⓐ in ADLs) changed to Ⓘ in ADLs.

Pt. shows excellent rehab potential to return home to live with spouse safely after 1 more week of treatment. Pt. would benefit from continued work on balance and activity tolerance, long-handled sponge and bath bench and instruction in use, as well as home eval and design home exercise program.

P: One additional week of b.i.d. treatment is requested in order to work on ↑ balance and activity tolerance needed for Ⓘ in ADLs, and to complete home eval, design home exercise program.

Worksheet 8-4

Reevaluation Report

Using the following checklist, determine whether the note on the preceding page meets the standards for reevaluation reports.

CRITERIA	COMPLIANCE
What tests were readministered and were the results reported?	
How do the current findings compare to the previous results?	
What are the changes in anticipated functional outcomes?	
What revisions are being made in the goals, objectives, and interventions?	
What revisions are being made in the frequency and duration of treatment?	

Adapted from Elements of Clinical Documentation *(Revision) (Thomson & Foto, 1995)*

Discharge Summaries

Occupational therapy treatments are discontinued by the OT when it is determined that either the patient's goals have been achieved, the patient has received maximum benefit from therapy, or the patient is transferred to another facility (Hirama, 1996). According to the *Standards of Practice for Occupational Therapy* (AOTA, 1998) an OTA may make recommendations to the supervising OT that a patient's therapy be discontinued and may also contribute to the discharge process under the OT's supervision, depending on the level of experience of the OTA.

A discharge summary (also called a discontinuation report) is used to summarize the course of a patient's treatment and to make recommendations for referral or follow-up care. Discharge notes often follow a format of their own, stating why and when the patient was referred, giving a summary of the initial findings, the course of treatment followed by a summary of progress, and any recommendations for follow-up care.

Given the time constraints and productivity standards common in practice today, you might wonder why a therapist would spend valuable time writing a note on a patient who is no longer on the caseload. Typically there are several reasons to justify the use of time in this way. First, the patient may be discharged to a less restrictive level of care rather than to home, and from one therapist to another while still requiring treatment. For example, a therapist providing acute care might discharge a patient to the therapist who is providing rehab care. The therapist doing rehab care then discharges the patient to the therapist providing home health care. Ideally, each therapist is able to use the discharge summary to build on skills developed under the previous therapist's care.

Even if the patient is discharged home or to a situation that does not include further occupational therapy services, the patient may need to be readmitted at a later time. If the OT receives a referral on a readmitted patient who was not previously on her caseload, it is very helpful to know what was done, what gains were made, and how the patient responded, along with what worked and what did not. In some cases, the doctor who made the referral may be the only follow-up available for the patient. In addition to providing follow-up care to his patient, he may want to know how his referral for occupational therapy was handled, what benefit has accrued to his patient, and whether to use occupational therapy in the future.

According to *Elements of Clinical Documentation* (Revision) (Thomson & Foto, 1995), discharge summaries should contain a summary of the course of treatment, including the number of treatment sessions and the consumer's response. The goals and objectives are examined to see whether they were achieved, fully or partially. Current functional status is compared to functional status prior to therapy. Any home programs and follow-up plans are noted, and recommendations and referrals are made. Under the supervision of an OT, an OTA may contribute to the discharge process. In some instances, to fulfill federal and state regulations, discharge notes written by an OTA should be co-signed by the OT to demonstrate that adequate supervision has been provided (Pinson, 1998). Again, it is important to determine what the requirements are in your own state and facility and abide by those guidelines.

Discharge summaries may be done as SOAP notes, or the facility may have a particular form or format that is to be used. We will be evaluating one that is in a SOAP format and a one that is done on a facility form. Some facilities use the same form for admission and discharge, making it quicker to prepare the discharge report.

Read the following discharge summaries and use Worksheets 8-5 and 8-6 to determine whether these summaries meet the AOTA criteria.

Hospital and Rehabilitation Center Discharge Summary

Date: 2/19/00 Time: 9:00 AM

S: Resident said, "I feel so much better than I did a while back. I feel like I've come a long way."

O: Resident seen for discharge planning from Medicare A → Medicare B. Resident seen 15/20 tx sessions from SOC. Resident illness prevented attending 5 sessions. Resident seen for ADL retraining, toileting, functional transfer training, ↑ AROM and strength.

Resident level of function at D/C as follows:

Goals:	Initial:	D/C:
Dressing UE Ⓘ	Min Ⓐ for balance	Set-up
Dressing LE Ⓘ	Mod Ⓐ for balance	Set-up c̄ CGA for standing to don pants and panties
Bathing UE Ⓘ	Min Ⓐ	Ⓘ UE
Bathing LE Ⓘ	Min Ⓐ	Ⓘ using long-handled sponge

Transfers		
Sit ↔ supine Ⓘ	SBA	SBA
Sit ↔ stand Ⓘ	Min Ⓐ	SBA
Stand ↔ w/c or toilet	CGA c̄ mod verbal cues	SBA
	Shoulder abd-65° (strength 2)	Shoulder abd 90° (strength 3)
AROM-WFL	Shoulder flex-55° (strength 2)	Shoulder flex-60° (strength 3)
	Elbow-0-125 (strength 3-)	Elbow-WFL (strength 4)

A: Resident exhibited an increase in AROM and strength. Resident has met bathing and hygiene goals. Dressing and transfer goals partially met. Resident is continuing to make progress and would benefit from further OT intervention to ↑ UE strength and activity tolerance to perform ADLs Ⓘ and meet all goals.

P: Discharged from skilled OT 2° change of status from Medicare A → Medicare B. Request physician's orders to reevaluate under Medicare B. Upon physician's orders, recommend skilled OT intervention 3x/week to increase activity tolerance and strength to perform ADLs Ⓘ.

Worksheet 8-5

Discharge Summary #1 (SOAP Format)

Use this worksheet to determine whether the preceding discharge summary meets the AOTA criteria.

Criteria	Compliance
What interventions were used?	
How many treatment sessions were there?	
How did the consumer respond?	
To what degree were the short- and long-term functional goals achieved?	
How does functional status prior to therapy compare to status at discharge?	
Is there evidence that a home program was or was not given? Is it attached?	
What is schedule and specific plan for follow-up?	
What are the recommendations pertaining to the consumer's future needs?	

Adapted from Elements of Clinical Documentation *(Revision) (Thomson & Foto, 1995)*

Rehabilitation Center Occupational Therapy

Discharge Summary

Date: 2/25/02 Time: 3:00 PM

Course of Rehabilitation

Pt. seen 20/20 sessions from SOC on 1/25/02. Skilled instruction in adaptive techniques for ADLs provided. Pt. progress was good and she met all tx goals. Pt. now requires SBA in all transfers, lower body ADLs, upper body ADLs, grooming/hygiene. She is Ⓘ in toileting. Pt. also requires SBA in feeding after set-up. Dressing from armchair with wheeled walker, set-up only but SBA for standing and to pull pants up over hips. Bathing is SBA with min Ⓐ w/c ↔ shower using tub bench.

Patient Education

Recommendations for additional adaptive equipment and modifications to home discussed with pt. and caregiver. Pt. and caregiver were instructed in home exercise program of theraband, free weights, wands, and other activities to choose from for Ⓑ UE strengthening. HEP discussed with pt. Pt. demonstrated ability to perform exercises correctly (refer to attached HEP).

Discharge Recommendations/Referrals

Discharge with home caregiver. Continue home exercise program. Assistive equipment recommended: walker basket and reacher holder for walker. Pt. already has wheeled walker, reacher, dressing stick, sock aid, long shoehorn, and functional bathroom equipment, and has demonstrated ability to use these correctly and safely. Pt. will be seen in outpatient PT. No direct occupational therapy services are recommended at this time.

Paul Howard

Worksheet 8-6

Discharge Summary #2 (Facility Form)

Use this worksheet to determine whether the preceding facility discharge summary meets the AOTA criteria.

Criteria	Compliance
What interventions were used?	
How many treatment sessions were there?	
How did the consumer respond?	
To what degree were the short- and long-term functional goals achieved?	
How does functional status prior to therapy compare to status at discharge?	
Is there evidence that a home program was or was not given? Is it attached?	
What is schedule and specific plan for follow-up?	
What are the recommendations pertaining to the consumer's future needs?	

Adapted from Elements of Clinical Documentation *(Revision) (Thomson & Foto, 1995)*

Chapter Nine

Documentation in Different Practice Settings

In this chapter we will examine documentation practices in three different practice settings: mental health, public schools, and long-term care facilities. Each of these has some requirements that are specific to the setting or the primary payment source. Documentation for these settings is different in some ways from the examples you have learned so far.

Documentation in Mental Health

If your first job is in a mental health setting, you might think that nothing you have been taught about documentation applies. Problems, goals, and interventions are often multidisciplinary and may be written in a different format from what you have learned. The language used in the documentation will seem less specific. Also, intervention is provided in a milieu environment involving a multitude of mental health professionals all working toward the same goals with the patient. Occupational therapy services are often included in a treatment service designated as adjunctive therapy, activity therapy, or expressive therapy that may include therapeutic recreation specialists, music therapists, art therapists, and dance therapists. The roles often overlap and there is a blurring of professional identities. The reimbursement is usually not discipline specific in these types of settings, and therapy services are usually inclusive in a room rate for the facility.

One of the exceptions is geriatric psychiatric mental health units or partial hospitals where the patients are usually insured through Medicare. The documentation is similar to inpatient Medicare requirements but the types of intervention covered include psychiatric occupational therapy services as well as self-care interventions (Lopes, 1998). As occupational therapy services become more community-based, the reimbursement patterns change and the funding may not be client specific but service specific. The documentation may be based more on program outcomes and population-based services (Ramsey & Auerbach, 1997). Even so, the documentation of services provided in community-based programs should reflect the principles and concepts used for occupational therapy assessments, plans of intervention, and records of progress of recipients of services. This means that your documentation should be objective and measurable and focused on occupational performance.

Initial evaluation reports often reflect the disciplines included in activity therapy rather than each discipline, thus losing some of the professional identity of occupational therapy. From the initial evaluation, the occupational therapist contributes to the treatment team's efforts to compile a list of problem statements.

Multidisciplinary Treatment Plans in Mental Health Care

Treatment plans in mental health are usually multidisciplinary. The therapeutic milieu is considered to be critical in caring for patients who have mental illnesses, and the individualized treatment plan (ITP) in a mental health setting is a contract for change between the patient and all members of the treatment team. After each individual discipline assesses the patient's needs and strengths, the team meets to formulate a list of the problems to be addressed. From this problem list, each individual discipline suggests goals, objectives and interventions for treatment within that discipline. All goals, objectives, and interventions for each discipline involved in the patient or client's care are written into one comprehensive plan.

If major problems or concerns have been identified in the evaluation, they must be documented somewhere on the ITP. It is critical that the plan is formulated by all who will be participating in it including the client and all staff who will be providing any part of the treatment. Multidisciplinary plans can often be quite long, since they are compilations of several different disciplines. These plans are similar to those developed by teams in a rehabilitation or school setting, but differ in that all staff are working toward the same goals through different interventions.

The plan must be easily understood by the patient or client and there must be some indication that the patient is in agreement with the plan, as required by most accrediting agencies. This is usually accomplished by the patient's signature on the bottom of the plan.

A multidisciplinary plan may contain fewer objectives per goal than a discipline specific plan. Success in writing a multidisciplinary treatment plan depends on:

- The involvement of the client (and family, if they are a part of the client's present life).
- The willingness of each member of the treatment team to cooperate in a coordinated effort to carry out specific interventions.
- Regular evaluation of the effectiveness of the plan and changes in direction in interventions that have not been effective.

Functional problem statements in a mental health practice setting are traditionally divided into two parts, as noted in *Chapter One*. The problem itself is stated in one or two words, such as "depressed mood," "noncompliant behavior," "suicidal ideation," or "alcohol withdrawal." The behavioral manifestations that follow give the performance areas and performance components. For example:

Problem: Chemical dependence

Behavioral manifestations: Mark has been using alcohol since age 12 with increasing frequency over the last year, and also admits to using cocaine, "crystal," opium, and marijuana; resulting in a failed marriage, loss of two jobs, and involvement with the criminal justice system.

Problem: Drug use

Behavioral manifestations: Kathy uses marijuana on a daily basis until she becomes high; resulting in depression and verbal altercations at home and in school.

Problem: Noncompliant behavior

Behavioral manifestations: Patient disobeys foster parents by running away, refusing to follow rules or requests, and engaging in sexual activity; resulting in six foster home placements in the past 4 years.

Problem: Suicide risk

Behavioral manifestations: During the week prior to admission, the patient verbalized suicidal ideation, stating that life was no longer worth living. On the day of admission he purchased a handgun.

Goals and **objectives** are often interdisciplinary, contributing to the role diffusion and lack of professional identity. Each discipline works on the same goals, using its individual treatment strategies. Occupational therapists in an inpatient mental health practice setting must decide what constitutes an instrumental ADL. Answering this question is one of the challenges of working in a setting that requires the team to document its ability to work together to provide a therapeutic milieu. Is remaining sober, decreasing family conflict, or keeping a marriage together an IADL? In addition, goals and objectives are often selected from computer programs or provided on preprinted sheets for each problem. In community settings, occupational therapy goals can be related more easily and clearly to ADL functioning.

Interventions are usually focused on the goals of the milieu setting, and those specific to activity therapy may be addressed by activity therapy in general and not specific to the disciplines represented by the activity therapy staff. The choice of interventions may depend largely upon what treatment groups are being provided by the facility, with the ability to individualize intervention strategies within the groups themselves. Selecting meaningful treatment interventions can be an interesting challenge. For example, most patients may attend communication groups, but within those groups, you as an OTA are able to customize the way you choose to increase communication skills for each individual patient. A good therapist learns to individualize goals for each patient in the group while still providing for the needs of the group as a whole.

When planning treatment, the client's assets (good verbal skills, intelligence, etc.) will be the tools that the client has to use in overcoming her problems. A "strength" in this context is an ability, a skill, or an interest that the client has used in the past or has the potential for using. Assets can include such things as the client's interests (enjoys playing music), abilities (writes well), relationship skills (has a good relationship with her father), and social support systems (minister keeps in contact). Assets may also be past abilities that the treatment team wants to encourage as treatment progresses (Jane was physically active before she became ill). Some interests (enjoys going to bars on weekends) may not be assets.

Behavioral Health Center Master Treatment Plan

Name: Tina W. **Date:** 12/27/01 **Page:** 1
Problem #: 1
Problem: Tina states that she does not have any good feelings about herself and that she has considered suicide, resulting in safety concerns.

Goal: Tina will verbalize both positive feelings about herself and the absence of suicidal ideation by D/C on 1/31/02.

Start Date	Measurable Objectives	Exp. Date Achieved	Method of Treatment	Freq.	Responsible Person
12/27/01	Tina will identify areas of her life that she feels are inadequate and discuss with primary therapist	12/30/01	Individual therapy	2x wk	S. Young, MEd
12/27/01	Tina will identify five areas about herself that are positive and discuss in groups and in individual therapy	1/7/02	Individual therapy Discussion with nursing staff Occupational therapy Emotions Anon.	2x wk Daily 3x wk 3x wk	S. Young, MEd A. Smith, RN S. Matsuda, COTA A. Smith, RN
12/27/01	Tina will discuss areas of her life that are positive and negative with peers and receive feedback in group therapy, Emotions Anon., and OT	1/14/02	Group therapy Emotions Anon. Communication skills group Step study	5x wk 3x wk 1x wk 3x wk	P. Alton, MEd A. Smith, RN S. Borcher, OTR S. Williams, BSW
12/27/01	Tina will select three new activities that she feels would be beneficial to her life and compose a plan for continuing these after d/c	1/20/02	OT will introduce Tina to a new leisure skill	3x wk	S. Matsuda, COTA
12/27/01	Tina will discuss her needs, assets, and plans with her mother	1/20/02	Individual therapy to formulate list of needs and a plan Family therapy to discuss plans and needs with mother	2x wk 1x wk	S. Young, MEd S. Young, MEd
12/27/01	Tina will complete all school assignments and earn passing grades in all subjects	1/30/02	Education staff will provide positive feedback for good schoolwork	5x wk	M. Green

Behavioral Health Center Master Treatment Plan

Name: Tina W. **Date:** 12/27/01 **Page:** 2
Problem #: 2
Problem: Tina expresses her anger at her mother by choosing the "wrong" boyfriend, lying, and running away, resulting in her removal from the home.

Goal: Tina will verbally express her anger to her mother by D/C on 1/31/02.

Start Date	Measurable Objectives	Exp. Date Achieved	Method of Treatment	Freq.	Responsible Person
12/27/01	Tina will attend health center groups that provide educational material on dealing with feelings	12/30/01	Psycho Ed. Emotions Anon. Occupational Therapy Group therapy	3x wk 3x wk 1x wk 5x wk	M. Eveker, RN A. Smith, RN S. Matsuda, COTA P. Alton, M.Ed.
12/27/01	Tina will discuss past ways of dealing with anger with primary therapist	1/7/02	Individual therapy	2x wk	S. Young, M.Ed.
12/27/01	Tina will list three alternate ways of dealing with her anger toward her mother	1/14/02	Appropriate way of dealing with anger will be discussed in individual therapy and OT	3x wk	S. Young, MEd S. Borcher, OTR S. Matsuda, COTA
12/27/01	Tina will practice alternative ways of dealing with her anger	1/20/02	All staff will remind Tina to practice her alternative methods when she becomes angry	Daily	A. Smith, RN S. Matsuda, COTA
12/27/01	Tina will enter into a behavior contract with her mother regarding how anger is to be expressed and received in their household.	1/20/02	Individual therapist will assist the family in writing the contract	2x wk	S. Young, MEd

Some mental health centers use prepackaged treatment planning sheets or mix-and-match computerized programs from which problem, goal, and intervention statements can be selected. In a mix-and-match program, the computer provides prompts from which the therapist selects the problem statements, goals, objectives, and treatment interventions that will be used for the individual patient.

When using prepackaged treatment planning sheets, the problems are expressed briefly (e.g., depressed mood, drug abuse, suicide risk) and the behavioral manifestations that apply to the individual patient are written in.

There is a list of long-term goals, or outcomes, such as these:

Patient will report the absence of suicidal ideation.

Patient will identify three new coping strategies to use when he feels the urge to use drugs.

All members of the interdisciplinary treatment team work on these goals while the patient is in the therapeutic milieu. The wisdom of using multidisciplinary goals without a strong functional component for occupational therapy practice has been seriously questioned by therapists who practice in mental health settings (Kannenberg, 1998). The question of exactly what constitutes an IADL in mental health care has not been definitively answered at this time.

On a prepackaged form there is a list of potential interventions that would also be addressed by the treatment team. Interventions might include such strategies as the following:

- Evaluate the patient.
- Encourage patient to express emotions.
- Teach new coping skills.
- Encourage the patient to verbalize alternatives to previous coping strategies.
- Assist the patient to develop a discharge plan that will prevent recurrence.

Each discipline implements the interventions in its own way. In relation to the five intervention strategies listed above, the OT does an occupational therapy evaluation to determine problems in occupational performance areas. As a part of the occupational therapy team, an OTA can participate in using media and groups to encourage the patient to express emotions, teach new coping skills and encourage the patient to verbalize alternatives. Social work adapts the same treatment interventions to individual and group therapy, and nursing implements the interventions on the unit. In this situation, there are sheets provided for each goal that are commonly used. It is individualized to the patient by stating behavioral manifestations of the problem, and by adding and deleting outcomes and/or interventions.

Treatment Notes

Formal treatment notes are rarely written in an inpatient mental health setting except when incidents, such as patient injury, occur and require documentation. One of the exceptions is geriatric psychiatric inpatient and partial hospitalization units where the patients are usually Medicare insured. In these settings, the documentation follows Medicare requirements.

Progress notes are usually written weekly, and an OT or OTA makes treatment notes for his own use in compiling the progress notes. However, if a patient with a mental health diagnosis is seen in home health, the Medicare standards for home health that require treatment notes for each visit apply.

When you begin thinking in the language of mental health, like "brightened affect," "less delusional," or "improved mood," it is easy to begin letting go of your ability to think in more objective and measurable terms. If you think about it, though, there are always clues that you are using to decide just exactly why you think the patient's affect is brighter or his mood is improved. Perhaps you are seeing him smile more frequently, or initiate conversation more often, or respond to your "hello" by making eye contact. Perhaps she takes less time to get up and dressed in the morning, or is more easily persuaded to attend OT. These indicators are all measurable, and it is very helpful to the treatment team if you are able to report your observations in measurable and behavioral terms.

The trend toward role diffusion is making it more difficult for OTs to document occupational therapy as a service that offers good value for the dollars spent in mental health care. As resources shrink and costs expand, we need to focus on documenting functional changes that are cost-effective and meaningful to both the payer and to the consumer. As noted in Chapter One, we are in the business of solving problems in occupational performance, and there are a myriad of occupational performance deficits present in the lives of people who have mental illness and chemical dependency. If we want to remain a viable force in inpatient mental health settings and if we want to continue to address the psychosocial issues related to physical dysfunction, we need to be able to document what we do that is unique. We need to be clear about the way our services change functional outcomes (Kannenberg, 1998).

An example of a progress note written by an OTA in a mental health setting follows. Notice that this note is specific and related to daily living skills.

Behavioral Health Center Occupational Therapy Progress Note

S: In assertion group on Tuesday 10/11/01, pt. talked about how her life had taken a "downward spiral" since early September, and she had become more passive and less proactive in getting her needs met, although she had not been aware of it at the time.

O: Pt. attended assertion group 2/2, communication group 1/1, and ADL group 3/5 this week. She was on time to 4/6 groups without reminders, wearing neatly pressed clothing, makeup, and an ornament in her hair. In assertion group on Thursday 10/12 she shared (without prompting) 2 stories about her usual way of dealing with retail situations. In communication group she spontaneously answered one question addressed to the group as a whole, and in ADL group she offered to assist another pt. with his checkbook.

A: Pt.'s spontaneous actions in groups and willingness to share verbally seem to indicate an improved mood this week. Her unprompted attendance is up this week from 2/8 to 6/8 groups. Her improved dress, hygiene, and makeup also indicate an improvement in mood from last week. Pt. would benefit from planning a structure for her days to prevent another "downward spiral" after discharge.

Goals #1 (assertion) and #2 (communication) are met as of this date.

Goal #3 (leisure skills) is continued through discharge on 10/19/01 pending formulation of a plan.

Goal #4 (ADL) was discontinued on 10/11/01.

P: Pt. to be seen in groups for 3 more days, with discharge anticipated on Wednesday of next week. ADL group will be used for preparing the structured plan for using her time. Pt. will prepare a plan including at least one planned activity per day for at least 5 days out of 7 after discharge and will discuss it with her husband and social worker by discharge on 10/19/01.

Critical Care Pathways in Mental Health

As length of stay has shortened for psychiatric diagnoses, some mental health settings have begun using critical care pathways as well as the standardized treatment planning programs discussed earlier. Critical care pathways in mental health are multidisciplinary and are conceptually the same as those in rehabilitation. The plan for the consumer's care for each day for each discipline is preplanned in order to make the most efficient use of staff time during the short length of stay, while still making sure the consumer's needs are met. Critical care pathways are discussed later in this chapter.

Documentation in School-Based Practice

When your caseload consists of children in the public schools, you learn a slightly different language for the same concepts. In this setting you will provide treatment based on a multidisciplinary plan called the IEP. The problems, goals, and interventions identified will focus on behaviors and skills the child needs in order to be successful in school. The IEP is compiled by therapists, teachers, and parents and deals specifically with the child's educational problems and needs. Based on an assessment from each discipline, it details the current problems, goals, and interventions for the child in all areas including occupational therapy for the current school year. The treatment principles and concepts are basically the same, only the language is different. That language difference, however, is very important.

Functional problem statements are exclusively problems of occupational performance in the educational setting, even though the child may have many deficits in other areas of life.

Goal statements are written for the duration of the school year, rather than using a timeline for each goal. In this setting, goals for the school year are called "objectives." Sometimes the format is slightly different, with "criteria" added to make the goal specific. It is very important not to set goals for performance components in this setting.

Interventions are specific to the educational setting as well, even though the child may also need treatment for problems in other areas of occupational performance.

Since an IEP can be quite long, the one provided here has been condensed from its original 26 pages to show only those aspects that are representative or most pertinent to occupational therapy.

Schools—Special Services Department

Individualized Education Plan

Student: Truman T.
Date of Birth: 9/17/89
Parents: Linda and Ellis T.
Teacher: Mary Ellen W.
Case Manager: Sharon Y.
IEP Conference Date: 5/23/99
Annual Review Date: 5/23/00
Duration of Services: 1 year
Initial Placement Date: 9/27/98

Service Model: Regular education: 100 minutes **initiated** 5/24/99 **ending** 5/24/00

Special Education: 1550 minutes **initiated** 5/24/99 **ending** 5/24/00

Related Services: Occupational therapy, physical therapy, adaptive PE, special transportation

Placement: Self-contained classroom

Assistive Devices: Glasses **Physical Education:** Adaptive PE

Special Transition Services Needed: Instruction, related services, daily living skills

Specialized Materials: Easel, bookstand for academic and fine motor activities, enlarged monitor for computer, pencil grip

Notification of Progress: Parents will be given a copy of the goals and progress four times per year with the report card.

Present Level of Performance: Truman has been diagnosed with cerebral palsy (quadriplegic), developmental delays, and visual difficulties. He wears glasses and needs written work enlarged. He has a history of ear infections and has bilateral PE tubes in place. Truman displays low muscle tone, with compensatory fluctuating increased tone upon movement. Fine motor skills are affected by spasticity noted in both arms on passive range of motion. Grip strength has improved, but bilateral tasks remain difficult due to poor lateral trunk control. He requires minimal to moderate assistance to hold his arms in different positions simultaneously. He requires moderate assistance to use scissors. His speech and language skills are commensurate with his intellectual functioning, in the mentally handicapped range of abilities. The WISC II suggests that his general information and verbal reasoning skills are at a 6 year age level. Nonverbal abilities are at about the same level. Truman shows difficulty with visual-spatial abilities, visual-motor integration, gross-motor production, and visual-perceptual processing. Vocabulary is low. He has a relative strength in short-term auditory memory and ability to sequence small bits of information. His ability to perceive patterns and relations is impaired, as is his neuropsychological processing of tactile stimuli. His adaptive behavior is below average. Current level of functioning is the 1.0-1.5 grade level. Reading comprehension and spelling ability are age equivalent 6-0, with math computation at an age level of 7-0. Adaptive functioning suggests an age equivalent of approximately 5-0 years. He is able to use a telephone in an emergency, look both ways before crossing the street, and get a drink of water from a tap unassisted. Progress has been made in adaptive functioning, but significant deficits remain in regard to toileting, dressing, functional mobility, and food preparation skills. No significant behavioral difficulties exist either at school or at home. Truman has limited interactions with peers, and limited participation in the regular classroom. He attends technology lab twice a week with a student aide. He works best on a 1-1 basis for 15 to 20 minute intervals in a situation where auditory distractions are limited.

1. **Annual Goal #1:** Truman will demonstrate responsibility for classroom assignments and homework.
   Implementer: Special Education Teacher
   - **Short-term Objective #1:** Truman will be responsible for homework in different areas of study at least 2 times weekly.
   - **Evaluation Procedure:** Observation

   - **Short-term Objective #2:** Truman will be responsible for taking notebook home and returning it the following day. Homework assignments consisting of spelling words, reading and math sheets, counting change, and time worksheets will be listed in this book.
2. **Annual Goal #2:** Truman will improve skills in adaptive physical education.
   Implementer: Adaptive PE teacher/paraprofessional
   - **Short-term Objective:** Truman will sit up.
   - **Evaluation Procedure:** Observation **Criteria:** Without being reminded for ½ hour

3. **Annual Goal #3:** Truman will use computers in the classroom and computer lab.
   Implementer: Special Education Teacher/Paraprofessionals
   - **Short-term Objective:** Truman will use computers with assistance.
   - **Evaluation Procedure:** Observation **Criteria:** 80% accuracy
4. **Annual Goal #4:** Truman will improve math skills.
   Implementer: Special Education Teacher
   - **Short-term Objective:** Given a clock dial, Truman will say the time to the 5-minute interval.
   - **Evaluation Procedure:** Daily work **Criteria:** 80% accuracy 3 out of 4 tracking days
5. **Annual Goal # 5:** Truman will improve fine motor for greater success with classroom related activities.
   Implementer: OTA
   - **Short-term Objective #1:** Truman will cut an 8" straight line within ¼" of line using adaptive scissors with minimal assistance to adjust grasp and paper position.
   - **Evaluation Procedure:** Daily work **Criteria:** 75% accuracy
   - **Short-term Objective #2:** Truman will type 10 spelling words on an adaptive computer keyboard using isolated index finger movements.
   - **Evaluation Procedure:** Daily work **Criteria:** No more than two errors
6. **Annual Goal #6:** Truman will increase visual motor skills for greater success in academic work.
   Implementer: OT
   - **Short-term Objective:** Truman will demonstrate good attention to task and visual motor skills in order to sort 15 small items.
   - **Evaluation procedure:** Observation **Criteria:** Within 90 seconds with minimal verbal cues and 75% accuracy
7. **Annual Goal #7:** Truman will exhibit increased functional motor skills in the school environment.
   Implementer: Physical Therapist
   - **Short-term Objective:** Sitting on a box, Truman will lean forward and sit upright picking up objects from the floor.
   - **Evaluation Procedure:** Observation **Criteria:** Eight times with 50% assistance from therapist after 10 consecutive sessions

Least Restrictive Environment: Self-contained special education classroom
Related Services: Occupational therapy, transportation, assistive technology, physical therapy
Will student be receiving services in school closest to home? __X__ yes _____ no
IEP services that cannot be provided in the regular classroom: Math, reading, written expression, listening comprehension, language, physical therapy, occupational therapy, transition
Factors for consideration of removal:

- Nature and severity of the disability
- Difficulty performing activity of daily living at an age-appropriate level
- Receptive/expressive language skills interfere with communication
- Easily distracted/frequently off task

Diverse learning style of the student

- Individualized instruction
- Increased drill/practice to master skills
- Additional time to complete task
- Requires highly structured small-group setting
- Immediate corrective feedback
- Positive rewards
- Lacks social/behavioral skills for participation in regular classroom
- Requires exposure to experiences not available in regular classroom

Inability to engage appropriately with other students

- Requires inordinate amount of teacher time
- Learning styles cannot be addressed in regular classroom
- Expressive language skills inadequate for classroom participation
- Receptive language skills interfere with academic progress

Occupational Therapy Evaluation/Progress Report

This 13-year-old male has received occupational therapy services throughout his school years with treatment most recently three times weekly for 45-minute sessions to work on improving fine motor and visual motor skills. Truman lives with his parents who are very supportive, active in his care, and motivated to see him succeed to his highest potential. He has many adaptations in his home to promote independence and assist caregivers.

Truman presents as friendly and kind, and wanting to please. He apologizes when he is unable to complete what is asked of him, although at times he will complain of being too tired to complete a task. He is very social and gets along with both peers and adults. Due to his cognitive limitations, standard testing would not give valid results. For this reason, observation of functioning has been used.

Fine Motor

Low muscle tone with moderate spasticity noted Ⓑ upon PROM. Elbows are contracted by calcium deposits to -30° Ⓡ and -40° Ⓛ. Truman is Ⓡ hand dominant. Grip strength Ⓡ is from 15-20# and Ⓛ from 8-16# in the past year. Truman has difficulty with Ⓑ tasks due to lateral trunk instability that requires use of one hand to stabilize himself. He has a hypersensitive startle reflex that kicks in when he feels like he is losing his balance. He has been working on dissociating arms so that he can use one for movement while the other is doing a different movement, and requires moderate assistance to do this. He is able to open a soda can after the seal has been broken with extra time given. He requires verbal reminders 75% of the time to use his Ⓛ arm to stabilize an object with one hand while manipulating it with the other. He requires moderate assist for scissor use and requires assistance to stabilize the paper. His arms become stiffened as he recruits all his muscle fibers to hold on to scissors and paper. Despite this, he has made great gains in scissor use over the past year.

Visual Motor/Visual Perception

Truman has severe visual problems and needs adaptive equipment to compensate for his visual deficits, including a large screen monitor and adaptive keyboard with the letters in alphabetical order. For future use, an adapted keyboard with enlarged letters in the regular order is recommended. He is able to use the mouse to move coins on the screen into a narrow slot with 75% accuracy.

Truman has a poor ability to track objects and poor ocular motor control. It is hard to tell what he can see, because he often guesses at responses. He is able to find objects in the classroom and to maneuver his wheelchair around obstacles. He has demonstrated great gains in visual motor paper and pencil skills, progressing from the inability to draw vertical and horizontal lines to the ability to copy circles, squares, and triangles with moderate assistance and dot-to-dot guides. Adapted equipment (vertical slant board and enlarged writing utensils) are needed for writing.

Gross Motor

Overall low tone with compensatory fluctuating increased tone upon movement. Specific exercises are performed daily as a part of adaptive PE.

Sensory Integration

No sensory defensiveness or unusual sensory behaviors.

Self-Help

- **Functional Mobility:** Able to wheel his chair within school environment with extra time.
- **Feeding:** He generally chooses finger foods but has demonstrated ability to use utensils with built up handles.
- **Toileting, Dressing (coat), Wheelchair Positioning:** Requires moderate assistance for these tasks. He is very private with his toileting and prefers males to assist him. He often slides forward in his wheelchair and has difficulty sitting upright and righting himself once he has leaned to the side. He would benefit from a wheelchair back that provides some lateral support and a cushion that will decrease the slide forward.

Summary

Truman has made great gains in fine motor strength and visual motor skills over the past year. Harrington rod placement greatly increased his ability to interact within the school environment. He seems motivated to succeed. Strengths include his supportive family, his motivation, his general good health, and emotional stability. Areas of concern continue to be his muscle weakness with compensatory abnormal movement patterns and visual motor/visual perceptual difficulties. If daily strengthening continues to be provided by school staff, Truman would benefit from occupational therapy at a decreased rate to focus on monitoring and training staff to assist him with exercise, visual motor, and bilateral coordination tasks.

Recommendations

Continue occupational therapy services twice weekly for 45-minute sessions to work on areas of concern listed above. Continue use of adaptive equipment listed above. Begin transitional planning for skills necessary after high school.

Linda P. Eagle, OTR/L

Documentation in Skilled Nursing Facilities in Long-Term Care

Most residents who receive therapy services in long-term care settings at skilled nursing facilities are covered by Medicare, and documentation is usually done using specialized Medicare forms.

When a resident is first admitted, a multidisciplinary evaluation called the Minimum Data Set (MDS) is used to determine the level of care needed. For ease and efficiency, each discipline may be assigned a specific part of the MDS to complete. Facilities vary in how ADL sections are divided between occupational therapy and nursing. Residents are then divided into Resource Utilization Groupings (RUGs) according to how much care they need. If this process is done improperly, the resident will not be able to get the level of care needed. Also, inaccurate assessments and predictions about rehabilitation potential may result in the facility not being able to be reimbursed for care that is provided beyond what was indicated on the MDS.

The initial assessment for a Medicare Part B patient is recorded on a Medicare 700 form (Figure 9-1), and contains a history, any medical complications that will impact treatment, the reason for referral, and the level of function at the start of care. As you can see in the example that follows, there is very limited space available for recording the initial evaluation report. The treatment plan is divided into two sections. There is a small space to record "Plan of Treatment Functional Goals" (short-term goals) and the "Outcome" or long-term goals. There is a separate small space for interventions. The example that follows shows the information recorded in the amount of space that is available.

Progress notes are done monthly on a Medicare 701 form (Figure 9-2), which provides equally small spaces for the reason(s) for continuing treatment for an additional billing period. In this section goals must be clarified and the reason for continuing skilled occupational therapy must be documented.

OTs and OTAs working in skilled nursing facilities in long-term care settings must learn to be very concise, providing all the necessary information in the fewest words possible. Some therapists have learned to manage the space constraints by using a specialized computer program that contains the form and reduces the font to the smallest size that is readable. However, some therapists are in situations in which they need to hand write the information into the space provided while still recording everything that is required.

The Critical Care Pathway

In response to the changing health care payment systems, many facilities have developed a form of a standardized treatment plan called a "critical care pathway." Certain kinds of illnesses, surgeries, and disabilities follow a predictable course of recovery. The body responds in a similar way to the condition, even though each person's experience will be unique. Critical care pathways are part of overall quality improvement efforts in health care facilities. In striving for quality care in the most cost-effective manner, the focus of health care is on the outcomes of that care and on the major components that are involved in the delivery of the care (AOTA Managed Care Project Team, 1996).

The goals of critical care pathways and the monitoring involved in quality improvement programs are to provide some predictability in outcomes, to establish a system of integrating care provided by a myriad of disciplines, and to allow for comparative analysis of treatment and treatment settings. The format of the pathways allows for monitoring a patient's progress on a comparative basis (AOTA Managed Care Project Team, 1996).

In addition to standardizing treatment and establishing checkpoints along a timeline, the use of a standard treatment plan also is more efficient by avoiding unnecessary time spent in rewriting basically the same treatment plan for routine treatment approaches. The standardized plan does allow for adaptations to accommodate individual patient differences, such as multiple diagnoses.

Critical care pathways are usually established to be multidisciplinary but may be specific to occupational therapy. In a setting like a skilled nursing facility that primarily has residents with Medicare insurance coverage, the treatment and patient education provided by each discipline is usually designed to be completed in an allotted number of days that is

DEPARTMENT OF HEALTH AND HUMAN SERVICES HEALTH CARE FINANCING ADMINISTRATION	Part A Part B	Other Specify	FORM APPROVED OMB NO. 0938-0227

PLAN OF TREATMENT FOR OUTPATIENT REHABILITATION (COMPLETE FOR INITIAL CLAIMS ONLY)

1. PATIENT'S LAST NAME XXXXXXXXXX	FIRST NAME XXXXXX M.I X.	2. PROVIDER NO. XXXXX	3. HICN XXXXX
4. PROVIDER NAME Provident Rehabilitation	5. MEDICAL RECORD NO. *(Optional)*	6. ONSET DATE 3/23/02	7. SOC. DATE 5/5/02
8. TYPE: ☐ PT ☐ OT ☐ SLP ☐ CR ☐ RT ☐ PS ☐ SN ☐ SW	9. PRIMARY DIAGNOSIS *(Pertinent medical DX)* pneumonia, Parkinson's Disease	10. TREATMENT DIAGNOSIS Decrease in function 780.9	11. VISITS FROM SOC.

12. PLAN OF TREATMENT FUNCTIONAL GOALS GOALS *(Short-Term)* 2 wks: Pt. will be: 1. SBA in bed mobility with adaptations to use bedside commode. 2. Ⓘ c̄ sit↔stand transfers to bed and toilet. 3. Able to ambulate using walker with SBA for safety↔bathroom. 4. Propel self in w/c Ⓘ ½ way to dining room. 5. Min Ⓐ dressing. OUTCOME *(Long-Term)* 6 wks: In order to perform ADLs at home, pt. will be: 1. Ⓘ in mobility & transfers. 2. Ⓘ in toileting using bedside commode or bathroom. 3. Ⓘ in w/c mobility. 4. Ⓘ in dressing and bathing c̄ set-up.	PLAN ADL retraining Transfer training Functional Mobility training Safety education
13. SIGNATURE *(professional establishing POC including prof. designation)*	14. FREQ/DURATION (e.g. 3/wk x 4 wk) 5/wk x 2 wk then 3/wk x 4 wk
I CERTIFY THE NEED FOR THESE SERVICES FURNISHED UNDER THIS PLAN OF TREATMENT AND WHILE UNDER MY CARE N/A	17. CERTIFICATION FROM 5/5/99 THROUGH 5/30/99 ☐ N/A
15. PHYSICIAN'S SIGNATURE | 16. DATE	18. ON FILE (Print/type physician's name)
20. INITIAL ASSESSMENT *(History, medical complications, level of function at start of care. Reason for referral)*	19. PRIOR HOSPITALIZATION FROM TO ☐ N/A

Pt. is 73 y/o/f who lived alone and did accounting work until hospitalized for pneumonia 3/23/99 and transferred to this facility 5/1/99. Pt. states she wants to move to her daughter's home and be Ⓘ in transfers and mobility as in the past. Medical Hx. and complications include Parkinson's disease and frequent falls. Prior to her illness, pt. was Ⓘ in bed mobility, ADLs, meal & tax preparations. Pt. was referred by nursing on 5/5/99 2° to pt. feeling better and being able to benefit from therapy. Cognition: alert and oriented x3; uses phone to direct family and clients from bed. ADL tasks: Pt. mod Ⓐ in bathing and dressing due to fatigue from illness and complications of inactivity and Parkinson's disease. Pt. feeds self after set up. Mobility: Pt. max Ⓐ in bed mobility supine to sit; mod Ⓐ in transfers and requires SBA assistance to ambulate in room using wheeled walker for safety and is propelled in w/c outside her room by staff due to fatigue, balance and ambulation difficulties. AROM is WFL but pt. is slow to initiate movements. Strength is 4/5 in Ⓑ UEs. Grip strength is 10# on Ⓡ, 8# on Ⓛ. Pt. is motivated and rehab potential is excellent for discharge to daughter's home with caregiver and possible home health or meals-on-wheels assistance. Pt. would benefit from skilled OT instruction in safe use of assistive devices, transfer techniques, and home evaluation before discharge.

21. FUNCTIONAL LEVEL *(End of billing period)* PROGRESS REPORT ☐ CONTINUE SERVICES OR ☐ DC SERVICES

22. SERVICE DATES
FROM THROUGH

FORM HCFA-700 (11-91) Form 2701/3P BRIGGS, Des Moines, IA 50306 (800)247-2343 PRINTED IN U.S.A.

Figure 9-1. Department of Health and Human Services Health Care Financing Administration Form HCFA-700.

DEPARTMENT OF HEALTH AND HUMAN SERVICES HEALTH CARE FINANCING ADMINISTRATION	Part A	Part B	Other Specify	FORM APPROVED OMB NO. 0938-0227

UPDATED PLAN OF TREATMENT FOR OUTPATIENT REHABILITATION *(COMPLETE FOR INTERIM TO DISCHARGE CLAIMS. PHOTOCOPY OF HCFA-700 OR 701 IS REQUIRED)*

1. PATIENT'S LAST NAME XXXXXXXXXX	FIRST NAME XXXXXX · M.I X.	2. PROVIDER NO. XXXXX	3. HICN XXXXX
4. PROVIDER NAME Provident Rehabilitation	5. MEDICAL RECORD NO. *(Optional)*	6. ONSET DATE 3/23/02	7. SOC. DATE 5/5/02
8. TYPE: ☐ PT ☐ OT ☐ SLP ☐ CR ☐ RT ☐ PS ☐ SN ☐ SW	9. PRIMARY DIAGNOSIS *(Pertinent medical DX)* pneumonia, Parkinson's Disease	10. TREATMENT DIAGNOSIS Decrease in function 780.9	11. VISITS FROM SOC.
	12. FREQ/DURATION (e.g. 3/wk x 4 wk)		

12. CURRENT PLAN UPDATE, FUNCTIONAL GOALS *(Specify changes to goals and plan)*

GOALS *(Short-Term)*
2 wks: Pt. will: 1. be Ⓘ sit → stand transfers ↔ bed, toilet, and bedside commode. 2. Be CGA for balance after set-up in managing clothing during dressing bathing and toileting. 3. Demonstrate safe transfers and mobility with SBA from caregiver during home eval.

OUTCOME *(Long-Term)*
4 wks: In order to perform ADLs in her own home, pt. will be: 1. Ⓘ in mobility & transfers. 2. Ⓘ in toileting, dressing, and bathing c̄ set-up. 3. Ⓘ and safe in use of walker and w/c in facility & home.

PLAN
ADL retraining
Functional mobility
Safety education
Home Evaluation
Pt./Caregiver education

I HAVE REVIEWED THIS PLAN OF TREATMENT AND RECERTIFY THIS PLAN OF TREATMENT WHILE UNDER MY CARE

14. RECERTIFICATION
FROM 6/5/99 THROUGH 6/19/99 ☐ N/A

15. PHYSICIAN'S SIGNATURE	16. DATE	17. ON FILE (Print/type physician's name)

18. REASONS FOR CONTINUING TREATMENT THIS BILLING PERIOD *(CLARIFY GOALS AND NECESSITY FOR CONTINUED SKILL CARE)*

Pt. has made significant progress in 2 wks. as demonstrated in her ability to sit up in bed and to sit on the side of the bed with CGA using a trapeze bar, a firmer mattress and a small bed rail. Pt. is SBA c̄ sit ↔ stand transfers ↔ bed; ambulates using walker c̄ SBA for safety ↔ bathroom. Pt. propels self in WC Ⓘ in her room but requires staff assistance to go to dining room 2° to fatigue. Demonstrates good awareness of safety precautions by using brakes during transfers. Pt. progressed from mod to min Ⓐ in dressing and bathing but requires help managing clothing, doing fasteners, and bathing back when standing due to ↑ balance and AROM. Pt. would benefit from continued ADL retraining, transfer and mobility training using assistive devices, skilled instruction and a home evaluation of mobility and safety issues at home with caregiver assistance. Rehab potential is excellent for discharge to her own apartment in daughter's home in 4 wks.

19. SIGNATURE *(or name of professional, including prof. designation)*	20. DATE	21. ☐ CONTINUE SERVICES **OR** ☐ DC SERVICES

22. FUNCTIONAL LEVEL *(at end of billing period - relate your documentation to functional outcomes and list problems still present)*

23. SERVICE DATES
FROM THROUGH

FORM HCFA-701 (11-91) Form 2701/3P BRIGGS, Des Moines, IA 50306 (800)247-2343 PRINTED IN U.S.A.

Figure 9-2. Department of Health and Human Services Health Care Financing Administration Form HCFA-701.

established by the Diagnostic Related Grouping (DRG) system. An orthopedic unit in an acute care hospital may establish the number of days of treatment based on a retrospective analysis of the hospital's medical records of orthopedic hospitalizations and DRGs.

Critical Care Pathways in Rehabilitation

Some diagnoses, such as CVA, are too complex to use a standardized approach to treatment. Other diagnoses, such as a total hip replacement, are very compatible with the critical care pathway system. A critical care pathway for a patient with a total hip replacement resembles the following example:

Critical Care Pathways in Rehabilitation

Day One (admission to rehab, post-surgery)
- Initial evaluation
- Film on total hip precautions
- Review precautions and have patient demonstrate to ensure understanding

Day Two
- Skilled instruction in functional mobility while following hip precautions
- Assess, provide, and instruct in necessary adaptive equipment
- Begin upper extremity strengthening
- Begin ADL training (dressing, grooming, hygiene)

Day Three
- Continue UE strengthening
- Continue ADL training
- Skilled instruction in shower and tub transfers
- Introduce home program and have patient demonstrate to ensure understanding

Day Four
- Skilled instruction in car transfers and stair climbing
- Home evaluation for safety
- Reassess patient's understanding of home program

Day Five
- Discharge

Different Formats for Notes

Remember that SOAP is just a format—an organizational structure that may be used for any type of note. An initial evaluation can be written in a SOAP format, as can a treatment or progress note. There are other styles of notes that may be used instead.

Checklists, flow sheets, and other similar forms created by the facility are often used instead of SOAP notes to save time. These are an especially popular way to document an initial assessment because they allow quite a lot of information to be communicated with little time spent writing. The evaluation and discharge form presented in Chapter Eight was developed by Capitol Region Medical Center in Jefferson City, MO. It is a particularly good example because it covers a lot of areas in a small space without sacrificing the ability to individualize the information. It also documents the performance areas before the performance components, so that no time is wasted documenting performance components that do not impact function. Using the same form for both evaluation and discharge allows the reader to evaluate progress toward goals easily. There is ample space for comments so that the form can easily be individualized. Sometimes checklists or flow sheets are also used for treatment notes or progress notes.

Narrative notes are not formally organized into sections the way SOAP notes are organized. Narrative notes may present any information in any order desired. Good narrative notes usually contain the "A" data of the SOAP note. Narrative notes reporting primarily the "A" data are becoming more popular due to time and space constraints.

DAP notes are an adaptation of the SOAP format used in some facilities. In this format, the "D" (data) section contains both the "S" and the "O" information.

BIRP or PIRP notes are sometimes used in practice settings. Information in these format is distributed as follows:

B: The behavior exhibited by the patient.
I: The treatment intervention provided by the therapist.
R: The patient's response to the intervention provided.
P: The therapist's plan for continued treatment, based on the patient's response.

P: The problem/purpose of the treatment.
I: The intervention provided by the therapist.
R: The patient's response to treatment.
P: The progress and/or updated plan.

If you work in a facility that uses one of these formats, you categorize your information slightly differently than you do when you are writing a SOAP note.

Electronic Documentation

As we move into the 21st century, productivity standards have become more stringent, putting increasing demands on a therapist's time. As a result, we are beginning to see the use of more electronic documentation. This is bringing changes to the way we approach the documentation task, as well as to the format in which we write. For some, the ultimate electronic goal is a "single comprehensive, multiprovider lifelong health record" (Abdelhak, Grostick, Hanken, & Jacobs, 1996, p. 669). Before we get to this, however, there are many problems to be solved. The ease of access must be weighed against confidentiality. More tools must be developed. At present, we have a wide variety of niche products, many of which may be useful in occupational therapy practice. There are many software packages available to make our jobs easier and more efficient.

There are packages available to schedule our days as well as to send and receive mail, to evaluate patients, to compile treatment plans, to write notes, and to remind us when everything is due. Software packages for electronic systems offer us a menu from which to choose initial evaluations and to print the forms for recording the data. Other packages offer choices of problems, goals, objectives, and possible intervention strategies rather than requiring these to be compiled for individual patients. Such software can make our job simpler and save valuable health care dollars. However, there are pitfalls to be avoided in using electronic systems (Abdelhak, Grostick, Hanken, & Jacobs, 1996).

First, there is a temptation to interact solely with the computer in selecting goals, objectives, and treatment strategies, rather than including the patient in the process. This should be avoided, regardless of the extra time involved in setting goals and choosing intervention strategies with the patient rather than for the patient. Effective treatment requires the teamwork of the patient and therapist working toward mutually selected and agreed upon goals.

Secondly, there needs to be a way to individualize each section of the treatment plan or progress note. A good program will allow editing options or places for comments so that the documentation can be individualized to the patient. Medicare reviewers in the past have not looked favorably on "canned" plans and notes that were selected entirely from menus. One way to make an effective compromise between selecting from a menu and individualizing the statements is to use a mix-and-match system in which the menu offers components of the statement and allows the therapist to choose the components appropriate to the individual patient.

Finally, we need to make certain that the patient is our main focus, fitting the software to the patient's needs, rather than fitting the patient into the capabilities of the software package.

Chapter Ten

Making Good Notes Even Better

Now that you have learned to write effective SOAP notes, it is time to review your work and take your skills up to the next level. This chapter will contain a review of each of the SOAP categories, as well as a review of goals and intervention strategies. We will begin by determining what kind of information belongs in each category of a SOAP note.

Subjective

In this section you report anything significant the patient says about his treatment. If the patient is unable to speak, report on his nonverbal communication, if any. In the case of a young child, a confused patient, or a patient who is unable to communicate, you may use what the primary caregiver says. For example:

Patient reported that she bent to the floor to pick up her make up case this morning.

Patient's daughter reports that her mother is more alert this week.

Objective

Here you report your observations, either chronologically or in categories. This section begins with a statement of how long the patient was seen, where the patient was seen and the purpose for the session. It is written from the patient's point of view, focusing on the patient's response to the treatment provided, and de-emphasizing the treatment media. You should be specific about the assist levels. In this section you are professional and concise in your wording, using only standard abbreviations, and avoiding judging the patient. For example:

Resident seen for 45 minutes in dining room with daughter present for skilled instruction in maintaining hip precautions during household management tasks. Resident ambulated to dining room SBA for balance. Resident retrieved snack from refrigerator and utensils from drawer $\bar{c}$ SBA for safety. Resident required 4 verbal cues to remember hip precautions when stand → sit and when turning with walker. Resident able to retrieve items from floor after skilled instruction in using a reacher. Education provided to resident and daughter on hip precautions and safety during both basic and instrumental ADL tasks. Daughter stated that she understood and would help her mother remember.

Assessment

This is your professional opinion about the meaning of what you have just observed. In assessing your data, you will pay special attention to evidence of problems, progress, and rehab potential. The assessment ends with a statement of what the patient would benefit from. For example, in assessing the observation above, you might say:

Resident's inability to remember hip precautions during household management tasks without verbal cues puts her at risk for re-injury. Supportive daughter and ability to use adaptive equipment properly after instruction indicate a good potential for reaching stated goals. Resident would benefit from further skilled instruction in maintaining hip precautions during ADL tasks, sit ↔ stand, and transitional living skills.

Plan

Your plan contains a statement of how often and for how long you will be seeing the patient, your priorities and goals. For example:

Continue tx 3x wk for 1 wk to work on incorporating hip precautions into ADL tasks. Within 1 week pt. will be Ⓘ in IADL tasks following hip precautions 3/3 trials.

Worksheet 10-1

Soaping Your Note

Indicate beside each of the following statements under which section of the SOAP note you would place it.

_____ Pt. supine → sit in bed Ⓘ.

_____ Pt. moved kitchen items from counter to cabinet Ⓘ using Ⓛ hand.

_____ Problems include decreased coordination, strength, sensation, and proprioception in Ⓛ hand that create safety risks in home management tasks.

_____ Pt. reports that his fingers are stiff this morning and that he is having trouble handling small items like buttons.

_____ Pt.'s attention span is <5 minutes.

_____ Pt's ↑ of 15 minutes in activity tolerance for UE activities permits her to prepare a light meal Ⓘ.

_____ Child seen in OT clinic to work on fine-motor and visual perceptual skills.

_____ In order to return to work, pt. will demonstrate an increase of 10 lbs. grasp in Ⓛ hand by 1/3/02.

_____ Decreased proprioception and motor planning limit patient's ability to dress upper body.

_____ Continue tx daily for 2 weeks for retrograde massage to Ⓡ hand for edema control.

_____ Patient's correct identification of inappropriate positioning 100% of the time would indicate memory WFL.

_____ Patient reports that she cannot remember hip precautions.

_____ Pt. would benefit from further instruction to incorporate total hip precautions into lower body dressing, bathing, and hygiene.

_____ Learning was evident by patient's ability to improve with repetition.

_____ Pt. does not make eye contact during group session.

_____ Pt.'s request to take rest breaks demonstrates knowledge of her limitations in endurance.

_____ Pt. wrote bank check for correct amount to pay electric bill with 2 verbal cues.

_____ Pt. has progressed to a 3+ muscle grade of extension in Ⓡ wrist extensors this week.

_____ Pt. completed weight shifts of trunk x10 in each of anterior, posterior, left and right lateral directions in preparation for standing to perform home management tasks.

_____ Pt.'s appearance in mock interview indicates poor judgment and self-concept.

Worksheet 10-2

Subjective

Remember that the "S" or subjective section of your note contains the patient's perception of the situation. One common error made by new therapists in writing the subjective section of the note is that of simply listing anything important the patient had to say about his condition. In the example below, all the information is relevant, but does not form a coherent whole. This is not wrong, and is better than reporting irrelevant data. But it is less skillful than reporting an organized and coherent summary of what the patient had to say. Most of this patient's comments have to do with transfers. In the space below, write a more concise version of this "S."

Pt. told OTA she has real bad arthritis in her right shoulder and knee.
Pt. told OTA, "It hurts to stand on my leg."
Pt. stated "It [sliding board] needs to be moved further up on the seat."
When asked if she was ok after the transfer, she said "I'm just tired."
Pt. stated "I'm through" and requested help to get nearer the bed.
When pt. transferred to the bed, she said "This is the hardest part."
Pt. stated she prefers to approach transfers from the affected side.

S:

Writing the "O": Good Opening Sentences

When you first learned to write the "O" section of your note, you learned to show your professional skill in the first sentence. For example, suppose you are seeing a patient whose contractures are compromising his positioning. Instead of saying "Pt. seen for positioning." You might introduce your "O" by saying one of the following:

Patient seen bedside to educate caregivers on positioning to prevent skin breakdown.

Pt seen bedside to select positioning strategies to improve seated posture for mealtimes.

In another scenario, suppose you are doing some ambulation with a patient as a part of ADL activities. Since this might potentially be seen as a duplication of services with PT, you would need to be careful about the words you used. Instead of saying "Pt. seen for ambulation", you might say:

Pt. seen to increase dynamic balance and attention to Ⓛ UE for safety when ambulating around kitchen to prepare meals.

In the following worksheet, you will be given an opening sentence that could be changed to show how your professional skill is needed. Below the "old" opening sentence is information that tells you how the skill of an OTA was needed in the treatment session. Please rewrite the opening sentence to reflect how you bring your skill as an OTA to the treatment. Use the three examples above as a guide.

Worksheet 10-3

Writing Good Opening Sentences

Rewrite the following opening sentences to show how your skill as an OTA is important in this situation:

1. *Old opening sentence:* Patient seen for morning self-care activities.

   Information found later in the note:
   - Weight bearing precautions raise safety concerns during functional mobility.
   - Hip precautions result in limitations to Ⓘ performance of ADL activities and safe transfers ↔ toilet.
   - Pt. would benefit from skilled instruction in use of adaptive equipment.

2. *Old opening sentence:* Client seen at ACT to work on job skills.

   Information found later in the note:
   - Client demonstrates deficits in sequencing tasks, which ↓ his ability to work Ⓘ.
   - Bilateral coordination problems interfere with client completing an essential job function of opening/closing boxes.
   - Sensory registration deficits contribute to client's high distractibility during task completion.

3. *Old opening sentence:* Client seen for morning dressing.

   Information found later in the note:
   - Deficits include ↓ balance and ↓ bilateral motor control of upper extremities that ↓ ability to safely complete ADL activities and use a manual wheelchair for mobility.
   - Pt. would benefit from skilled education for safety in living at home.

4. *Old opening sentence:* Pt. seen in kitchen to work on Ⓘ in cooking.

   Information found later in the note:
   - Patient's problems include decreased dynamic standing balance and inattention of affected UE which raise safety concerns.

WRITING A COMPLETE AND CONCISE "O" – OBJECTIVE

In the objective section of your note, you report what you observed while providing treatment for the patient. As you gain skill, you become more aware of what to include and what to omit in order to be concise. Consider the following observation of a treatment session. What does it need to make it better?

Pt. was seen in room for further ADL training. Pt. participated in ADLs and transfer activities.

ADL

Pt. donned robe Ⓘ with set-up.

Pt. donned/doffed socks Ⓘ with set-up.

MOBILITY

Bed → chair with CGA.

Supine → sit Ⓘ.

This note does not have enough information. It is **too** concise. There needs to be some indication that skilled occupational therapy was provided. You could start with an opening sentence that shows why your skill as an OTA is needed in this situation. As it stands, it is apparent that someone observed the patient dress and transfer and recorded assist levels, but a rehabilitation aide or nursing staff could have done this. Secondly, the time required to do the activities documented in this note could be very short. If this is an hour treatment session, what else was done? If the patient was slow to do the things recorded above, what caused so few activities to take so long? Is there a cognitive problem? Is there a coordination, safety, or motor planning problem? Were adapted techniques or adaptive equipment used to allow the patient to be Ⓘ? Third, with this patient's documented level of independence, there is nothing in this note to justify further skilled occupational therapy. Unless this is the last session that will be provided, there needs to be information provided that will justify continued treatment.

Worksheet 10-4

Write a Complete and Concise "O" – Objective

Now it is your turn. Read the observation below. What does this note need to make it better?

Toilet transfers:	max Ⓐ
Toileting:	min Ⓐ with SBA 2° inability to support self with Ⓛ arm and to dress
UE dressing:	min Ⓐ, verbal cues, set up, Ⓘ in pulling shirt over head
LE dressing:	min Ⓐ pants to hips max Ⓐ pants to waist modified Ⓘ don Ⓛ shoe (elastic shoelaces) mod Ⓘ to don Ⓡ shoe
Ⓡ hand status:	Ⓡ fingers: small spasticity (index finger greatest amount) Thumb: cmc jt. painful in abd. & flex. Ⓡ wrist: flaccid

WRITING EFFECTIVE ASSESSMENT STATEMENTS

When OTAs are first beginning to write SOAP notes, it is sometimes difficult to decide what is an observation and what is an assessment. Anything you see a patient do is an observation. Its meaning in terms of your patient's ability to function in some performance area is your assessment. Sometimes the difference between an observation and an assessment is one of emphasis. You will assess other things than performance components. Often you will assess progress, potential to meet goals, and the emotional components of treatment. Remember that no new information may be introduced in the "A." This is an assessment of the data you have recorded in your observation.

In assessing performance components that are not within functional limits, you learned a formula that helps you be sure you have placed the emphasis correctly and have included all the necessary components.

Performance Component	Impact	Performance Area

It is not the only correct way to write assessments, but it will help you while you are first learning this skill. To assess a performance component not within functional limits, you will do the following:

- Determine the basic or core deficit (such as ½ AROM or inability to sequence).
- Make the deficit the subject of your sentence to give it the emphasis it needs in this section of your note.
- Decide whether the area of difficulty you have observed today is an indicator of a broader performance area. For example, is the decreased AROM you observed to be causing a problem in grooming also a problem in other basic ADL tasks? Will his inability to balance his checkbook also cause problems with other money management tasks? Do the problems you observed today put his safety at risk?
- Make certain your assessment statement tells how the problem areas impact the patient's life (performance area). After each problem you note (e.g. limited AROM, sequencing deficits, unstable balance), ask yourself "So what?" So he is unable to do that—what difference does it make? The answer to your "so what?" question is your assessment of the situation.

The following statements are examples of how an observation statement would be worded differently than an assessment statement. For example, suppose you are working with a patient who tells you she plans to return to living alone in her farmhouse. You have worked on teaching her some energy conservation techniques, but she forgets to incorporate these into her morning dressing routine. What is the basic or core problem for this patient? Why does it matter?

The following statement is an **observation** of the patient's behavior:

Pt. was unable to perform energy conservation techniques during morning dressing due to memory deficit.

However, phrased differently, it becomes an **assessment** of what was observed:

Memory deficit interferes with patient's ability to retain instructions in compensatory techniques such as energy conservation, which limits her ability to perform self-care tasks needed to return to prior (I) living situation.

Note that in the assessment statement, the OTA has identified the basic or core problem as the patient's inability to retain instructions she has been given. This might be followed by a recommendation to use memory cues of some kind. Otherwise, why should a payer continue to pay for instruction that will not be remembered? You might also want to consider her safety in living alone if her short-term memory is impaired.

According to the formula, the assessment does not repeat what was observed. Instead it begins with the performance component that is a problem, broadens the scope of the performance area to include related tasks, in this case all basic self-care tasks, and answers the question, "So what? Why does this matter in this patient's life?"

The following statement is an **observation** of what the OTA saw today:

Patient's problem-solving was functional and accurate with verbal prompts.

An **assessment** of the situation would sound like this:

Patient's need for multiple verbal prompts to solve social problems limits his ability to respond appropriately in unstructured social situations and to enter into successful relationships with others.

Note that in the observation statement, there was no performance area mentioned. In the assessment statement, you are addressing the performance areas that are impacted by his ↓ problem-solving skills.

This statement is an **observation** because it tells what the patient did:

Pt. tolerated vestibular and proprioceptive input well as evidenced by his choosing the activity.

Yes, his choosing the activity is an indication of his tolerance, and that is clinical judgment, but there are more important things to **assess**. One is his progress in tolerating input, and the other is the performance area impacted by this progress.

Patient's choices of activities with proprioceptive and vestibular components indicate progress in sensory tolerance necessary for attention to task in the classroom.

Worksheet 10-5

Differentiating Between Observations and Assessments

Identify which of these statements are observations and which are assessments. Remember that an observation will tell you what the patient did. An assessment will tell how the performance component that is a problem impacts a performance area.

_____ Pt. is unable to don AFO and shoe Ⓘ for ambulation.

_____ Inability to don AFO and shoe Ⓘ prevents pt. from ambulating safely around the house to live alone.

_____ Decreased sensory tolerance limits the patient's attention to task in the classroom.

_____ Patient requires verbal cues to stay on task due to decreased sensory tolerance.

_____ Patient was unable to incorporate breathing and energy conservation techniques, requiring several verbal prompts to complete task.

_____ Inability to incorporate breathing techniques and energy conservation techniques into basic ADL tasks s̄ verbal prompts limits her ability to live alone Ⓘ p̄ discharge.

The following statements are observations of something the OTA saw the patient do. Reword them so that they become assessments.

Patient demonstrated difficulty with laundry and cooking tasks due to memory and sequencing deficits.

A:

Patient unable to complete homemaking tasks or basic self-care activities independently due to decreased endurance and not following hip precautions.

A:

After use of behavior modification techniques, patient displayed courteous behavior for the remainder of the treatment session.

A:

Worksheet 10-6

Assessment and Plan

After you have written your observation of the treatment session, you assess the meaning of the data you have put in the "O." This is the heart of your note, and shows your critical thinking skills. You follow this with your plan for continued treatment. Write an assessment and plan for the following patient observation. Begin by making a note to yourself of the problems, progress, and rehab potential that you see. For any performance components not within functional limits, note the performance areas these performance components are likely to impact. Begin your plan by telling how often and for how long you will see the patient. Follow that with what you plan to do, and end with a goal.

O: Patient seen for 30 min. in OT clinic to work on functional movements of Ⓡ UE, dynamic sitting balance, and cognitive skills. Pt. needed mod Ⓐ in shifting weight to get to edge of w/c and max verbal cues to use correct posture and shift feet during standing pivot transfer w/c → mat. Pt. requires max verbal cues to initiate grasp of bag in beanbag activity. Pt. needs mod Ⓐ in reaching with Ⓡ UE. Pt. demonstrated ability to complete Ⓡ UE shoulder flexion required to toss bag approximately 2 feet with max verbal cues. Pt. demonstrated cognitive understanding of activity with mod verbal cues by stating desired goal to be achieved by accurate aim.

Problems/Progress:

Rehab Potential:

A:

P:

Worksheet 10-7

The "Almost" Note

This note is almost good enough. In fact, it seems quite good on the surface, but has major flaws in organization and clinical reasoning. This is a 78-year-old female who has had a Ⓛ CVA and has Ⓡ hemiparesis. What does this note need to make it better?

S: Pt. reports stiffness in Ⓡ hip, but improvement from previous pain. She states a preference for transferring to her left. Pt. states that she is willing to do "whatever it takes to get out of the hospital."

O: Pt. seen in room for work on dressing and functional mobility.

Transfer: Pt. SBA for standing pivot transfer bed → w/c to the left.
Pt. min Ⓐ with transfers w/c → toilet using grab bar.

Mobility: Pt. SBA with VC's to flex trunk when rolling from supine to Ⓡ side.
Pt. SBA supine → sit; min Ⓐ sit → stand.
Pt. Ⓘ in w/c mobility.

Dressing: Pt. Ⓘ in donning shirt.
Pt. min Ⓐ with VC's to don bra while standing.
Pt. Ⓘ in donning socks and shoes.
Pt. min Ⓐ with walker and VC in donning underwear and pants.
Pt. needs set-up for dressing activities.

UE ROM: Ⓛ UE — WFL.
Ⓡ UE — ↓ range in proximal shoulder flexion.

Static standing: Pt. CGA with walker Ⓑ UE support.

Dynamic standing: Pt. SBA with walker for balance.

A: Deficits noted in Ⓡ UE coordination, Ⓑ UE strength, and dynamic standing balance. Pt. Ⓘ in dressing EOB, but is min Ⓐ in dressing when standing with a walker. Ⓛ UE AROM is WFL but Ⓡ UE has deficits noted in shoulder flexion. Pt. needs SBA in bed mobility when rolling to unaffected side and min Ⓐ in sit → stand 2° ↓ UE strength. Pt. needs SBA for transfer to unaffected side in pivot transfer bed → w/c and min Ⓐ w/c → toilet. Pt. would benefit from skilled OT to continue UE strengthening and coordination exercises and to ↑ dynamic standing balance using walker, in order to ↑ Ⓘ in ADL's.

P: Pt. to be seen b.i.d. for 30-minute sessions to continue to work on dynamic standing balance. Pt. will require SBA in grooming activities standing sink-side with standard walker within 2 weeks.

Worksheet 10-8

Writing Functional and Measurable Goals

You know how to write goals and objectives using the FEAST method to insure that all the necessary components are present.

F: Function (If not embedded in the action)	For what functional gain?
E: Expectation	The patient will..?
A: Action	Do what?
S: Specific Conditions	Under what conditions?
T: Timeline	By when?

However, writing the components in that order sometimes leads to a very awkward sentence. Try rewriting the following goals in a more logical order, making sure that conditions are present in the goal statement.

Pt. will pivot while standing with SBA during toilet transfers in 1 day.

Pt. will be min Ⓐ in dressing UE and LE in 10 days.

Pt. will be min Ⓐ in toileting (dressing component) in 3 days.

Remember that you learned to de-emphasize the treatment media when you were writing your observation. This is also important in writing goal statements. Rewrite the following goal statements to emphasize the changes you would like to see in your patient's performance components and to de-emphasize the treatment interventions you are using.

Patient will place 8 ½-inch screws and washers on a block of wood with holes by 4/10/02.

Patient will make a clock using the appropriate materials while sitting by anticipated discharge on 5/12/02.

Client will stay in his chair without reminders and spend at least 30 minutes lacing the leather billfold during the 45-minute craft group session in 2 weeks.

Planning Treatment Interventions

As an OTA, one of your most important jobs is the generation of treatment interventions that will help the patient move toward his goals. Consider the patient described below:

Interventions to Interest Mr. Warren

Mr. Warren is a 54-year-old man who had a CVA and now has Ⓛ hemiparesis. He used to be an athlete, and is grieving the loss of the use of his left side. He has some proximal motion, and the OT wants him to use his left hand as a functional assist. This is her treatment note from last week:

S: Pt. reports that he is having problems using his Ⓛ UE and he prefers one-handed activities, saying "It won't work" and "I can't do it" when asked to use the Ⓛ UE as an assist. Pt. reports that he continues to perform the UE exercises he has been taught to maintain Ⓛ UE mobility.

O: Patient seen in room for skilled instruction in safe functional mobility during dressing activities and for strategies to incorporate Ⓛ UE into Ⓑ tasks as a functional assist.

Pt. CGA for balance while retrieving clothing from low drawers. Pt. incorporated Ⓛ UE into task by carrying clothing in Ⓛ axilla while using Ⓡ UE to hold cane for balance. Pt. SBA for balance and safety to retrieve hanging garment from closet using Ⓡ UE. Pt. able to maintain balance when spontaneously bending down to floor to retrieve dropped garment. Pt. able to verbalize two safe methods to transfer clothing to bed for set-up in dressing. Pt. min Ⓐ to use Ⓛ hand to stabilize small and medium sized bottles and Ⓡ hand to unscrew caps. Pt. tolerated ~5 minutes of reaching activity to retrieve bottles held @ various planes while sitting EOB. Patient demonstrated motion in the Ⓛ shoulder, but no active movement in Ⓛ wrist or hand.

A: Although pt. demonstrates good performance of one-handed techniques, he requires verbal cues and min Ⓐ to use Ⓛ UE as a functional assist. Progress is indicated by ↑ Ⓛ UE function proximally. Good rehab potential is indicated by patient's compliance with UE exercise program. Pt. would benefit from muscle re-education techniques for the Ⓛ UE, and further instruction in Ⓛ UE functional assist strategies during ADL activities.

P: Pt. to be seen daily for 1 more week in order to ↑ safety in functional mobility during ADL tasks, for muscle re-education in the Ⓛ UE, and for activities to ↑ use of Ⓛ UE as a functional assist in daily activities. Pt. will spontaneously use the Ⓛ UE as a functional assist for self-care activities at least 3 times in 10 minutes within 4 days.

Amanda Coughlin, OTR

Worksheet 10-9

Creative Treatment Interventions

You will be seeing Mr. Warren for the next week until he is discharged, and you want to find some interesting ways of incorporating his Ⓛ UE into functional tasks.

What is the short-term goal?

What interventions will you use? Remember, a goal is what the *patient* will do. Treatment interventions are what you will do to help him accomplish the goal.

Conclusion

Congratulations! If you have read all the material presented in this manual and completed all the exercises, you should be able to document your patient care to the most rigorous standards. The notes that follow are intended to provide you with examples of well-written notes from a variety of treatment settings. These examples, along with the ones included in the various chapters, should provide you with ideas for documenting some of the more common kinds of treatment sessions. If you work in a setting that is not represented, you are invited to contribute notes to the next edition of this manual.

We invite your comments, criticisms, ideas, and suggestions for ways to make this book better or more useful to instructors, students, and beginning OTAs. We also invite you to submit examples of documentation that you consider to be good examples of some particular concept (such as conciseness). We are particularly interested in notes that represent best practice in occupational therapy today.

When submitting a note, please include your name, address, and telephone number, along with your permission to publish the note. Please send your comments, suggestions, or notes to:

Sherry Borcherding/Carol Kappel
c/o SLACK Incorporated
Professional Book Division
6900 Grove Rd.
Thorofare, NJ 08086

The page that follows is a summary of everything you have learned about writing SOAP notes in occupational therapy. Pull it out and carry it with you to use as a quick reference guide while you are learning to document.

A Quick Checklist for Evaluating Your SOAP Note

Use the following summary chart as a quick reference guide to be sure that your note contains all the essential elements.

S (Subjective)

- ❑ 1. Use something significant the patient says about his treatment or condition.

O (Objective)

- ❑ 1. Begin this section with length of time, where, and for what reason the patient was seen.
- ❑ 2. Report what you see, either chronologically or using categories.
- 3. Remember to do the following:
  - ❑ De-emphasize the media
  - ❑ Specify what the part of the task the assistance was for
  - ❑ Show skilled occupational therapy happening
  - ❑ Leave yourself out
  - ❑ Focus on the patient's response
  - ❑ Avoid being judgmental

A (Assessment)

- ❑ 1. Look at the data in your "O" sentence by sentence, asking yourself what problems, progress, and potential you see.
- ❑ 2. Ask yourself "So what?" "Why is this important in the patient's life?" For each performance component not within functional limits, identify the impact it will have on a performance area.
- 3. End the "A" with "Patient would benefit from..."
  - ❑ Justify continued skilled occupational therapy
  - ❑ Set up the plan
    (Be sure the timelines and activities you are putting in your plan match the skilled occupational therapy you say your patient needs.)

P (Plan)

- ❑ 1. Specify how often the patient will be seen and for how long.
- ❑ 2. Tell what you will be working on during that time.
- ❑ 3. End with an LTG or STG, whichever is more appropriate for your patient and practice setting.

In Reviewing Your Note

- ❑ Make certain function is integral to the note. Also make certain everything goes together. For example, if you talk about inability to dress in the problem list, don't switch to feeding in the goals and showering in the plan.
- ❑ Remember to sign and date your note.

If you have read the text carefully you will know what each item means. For a more complete explanation, refer to the chapter that provides information in detail. There is a brief explanation of SOAP guidelines on the back of this sheet.

S (Subjective)

- Use something **significant** the patient says about his **treatment** or **condition**.
- If there is nothing significant, ask yourself whether you are using your interview skills to elicit the information about how the patient sees things.

O (Objective)

- Begin this section with length of time, where the patient was seen, and for what reason. For example:

  Pt. seen for 30 minutes bedside for functional mobility.
- Report what you see, either chronologically or using categories.
- Remember to do the following:
  - Focus on performance elements and de-emphasize the media.

    Pt. worked on tripod pinch using pegs.
  - When giving assist levels, specify the part of the task the assistance was for. For example:

    Pt. min Ⓐ for correct hand placement during pivot transfer to toilet.
  - Show skilled occupational therapy happening—make it clear that you were not just a passive observer.

    For example, don't just list all the assist levels and think that is enough.
  - Write from the patient's point of view, leaving yourself out.

    Pt. was positioned—rather than therapist postioned the pt.
  - Focus on the patient's response, rather than on what you did.

    Pt. able to don socks using dressing stick after demonstration.
  - Avoid being judgmental.

    For example, say he *"...didn't complete the activity."* Don't add *"...because he was stubborn."*

A (Assessment)

- Look at the data in your "O" sentence by sentence, identifying problems, progress, and rehab potential. Ask yourself what each statement means for the patient's occupational performance. This is your assessment of the data.
  - For example, if in your "O" you noted that pt. falls to the left when sitting unsupported, what do you think this means he will be unable to do for himself? For example:

    Pt. unable to sit EOB unsupported to dress.
- Be sure you have not introduced any new information.
- End the "A" with "patient would benefit from..."
  - Justify continued skilled occupational therapy.

    Pt. would benefit from skilled instruction in energy conservation techniques as well as continued work on AROM of the UEs, strengthening, and compensatory techniques for performing IADL tasks one-handed.
  - Set up the plan.

    Be sure the timelines you are putting in your plan match the skilled occupational therapy you document that your patient needs. For example, if you justify skilled occupational therapy by saying only *pt. would benefit from skilled instruction in energy conservation techniques,* then do not say that you plan to treat him twice a day for 2 weeks. Skilled instruction in energy conservation should take only one session, or at most 2 sessions.

P (Plan)

- Specify frequency and duration of treatment. For example:

  Continue tx one hour daily for 2 weeks.
- Identify the specific performance areas that will be addressed during that time.

  Pt. to continue OT one hour daily for 2 weeks for instruction in Ⓘ in bathing, grooming, and hygiene.
- End with a LTG or STG, whichever is more appropriate for your patient and the practice setting.

  By the end of the week, pt. will be able to don socks Ⓘ sitting EOB without losing balance.

Chapter Eleven

Examples of Different Kinds of Notes

This chapter provides examples of notes that would be written by an OT or OTA to document different stages of treatment in a variety of practice settings.

CONTENTS

The notes in this section were written by students, faculty, and practicing OTRs and COTAs. In most cases the signatures were omitted unless the person who wrote it wanted credit for his/her work, in which case the name has been used.

Initial Evaluation Report

Hospital and Rehabilitation Center
Initial Evaluation Report

Name: Rebecca B. **Age:** 80 **Date:** 5/3/01 **Time:** 8:30 AM
Primary Dx: Fx. Ⓛ hip **Secondary Dx:** HTN
Primary Payment Source: Medicare **Secondary Payment Source:** supplemental insurance
Admission Date: 5/2/01 **Estimated Length of Stay:** 4 days **Physician:** B. Garrett, MD
Pertinent History: Rebecca had gone upstairs to use the bathroom since there were none on the first floor. She became lightheaded, fell down the stairs and broke her hip. She was admitted for a total hip replacement yesterday. Her family lives out of town and cannot stay with her. She wants to return home.

S: Pt. stated that she would like to "get this leg well" and go home to "live a regular life." She reports living alone and being Ⓘ in all ADLs prior to admission.

O: Pt. seen in room for initial evaluation of morning ADL capabilities after THR. Pt. educated on use of ADL equipment for self-care tasks and adherence to hip precautions. Pt. demonstrated ability to repeat 2/4 hip precautions. During ADL evaluation pt. was observed flexing 8° to 10° beyond 90° and required four verbal cues to remain at or below 90° during the 45-minute session. Other three hip precautions were followed Ⓘ. Pt. able to complete sponge bath at sink after set-up for upper body, and used dressing stick with washcloth and verbal cues for lower body. Pt. able to bear wt. partially on Ⓛ leg; required min Ⓐ for balance with sit ↔ stand to bathe back peri area. Pt. able to complete upper body dressing after set-up. Pt. dons underwear and pants Ⓘ using a dressing stick. Pt. dons socks using sock aid after set-up with verbal cues. Pt. completes grooming tasks and oral care Ⓘ. Following verbal cues, pt. demonstrated good problem-solving by trying different body positions to perform ADLs while adhering to hip precautions and demonstrated understanding of adaptive aids by utilizing reacher and dressing stick correctly after instruction. Pt. demonstrated ↓ ADL tolerance as she required four 2-minute rest breaks during dressing tasks. Pt. then seen in OT clinic for physical evaluation.

Ⓑ UE AROM—WFL	Ⓑ UE strength—WFL
UE sensation-intact	Grip strength Ⓡ 47#, Ⓛ 43# (Ⓡ hand dominant)
Tripod pinch Ⓡ 10#, Ⓛ 5#	Lateral pinch Ⓡ 10#; Ⓛ 5#

A: Pt. demonstrated good motivation, problem-solving skills, and understanding of equipment use. Upper body strength and AROM were WFL, all of which indicate excellent rehab potential. Pt. is able to complete grooming tasks and oral care Ⓘ but is unsafe to complete lower body dressing and bathing due to ↓ activity tolerance, balance, and inconsistent compliance with hip precautions. Problem areas include ↓ balance in sit ↔ stand, ↓ ADL activity tolerance, and ↓ safety in ADL tasks. These problem areas negatively impact pt.'s ability to be Ⓘ and safe in ADL tasks. Pt. would benefit from skilled instruction on hip precautions and use of adaptive equipment with ADL performance, therapeutic activities that facilitate dynamic standing balance and ↑ ADL activity tolerance. Exploration of interim living arrangement or possible continued home visits and home equipment procurement if progress warrants discharge to home.

P: Pt. to be seen b.i.d. for 1 hour the next 3 days to ↑ Ⓘ in self-care tasks through instruction on hip precautions and use of adaptive equipment, with tasks to ↑ activity tolerance, and balance activities using reaching patterns while standing.

LTGs**:** By discharge (5/7/01) pt. will:

1. Safely complete lower body dressing and bathing modified Ⓘ utilizing adaptive equipment with 100% adherence to hip precautions.
2. Be Ⓘ and safe in toileting using adaptive equipment of walker and bedside commode.

Treatment Plan

Name: Rebecca B. **Age:** 80 **Primary Dx:** Left hip fracture/THR
Strengths: UE strength and AROM; intact cognition and motivation to return home.

Functional Problem: Unsafe in ADL tasks due to ↓ compliance with hip precautions following THR, ↑ fatigue, ↓ endurance for ADL tasks requiring frequent rest breaks.

LTGs: By discharge (5/7/01) pt. will safely complete LE dressing and bathing utilizing adaptive equipment with 100% adherence to hip precautions.

STG (By 5/5/01 pt. will:)	Interventions
1. Pt. will be able to complete basic ADL tasks while standing for 5-minute increments and taking rest breaks as needed by discharge date 5/10/01.	1. Instruct and have pt. verbalize 4/4 hip precautions.
2. ↑ ADL tolerance as demonstrated by not more than one 15 sec. rest break during dressing task of donning slacks.	2. Instruct in use of adaptive techniques/devices followed by demonstration of use in dressing and bathing activities.
3. Safely bathe her peri area utilizing adaptive techniques and devices with 100% adherence to hip precautions.	3. Educate pt. & provide written instructions on energy conservation techniques. Evaluate understanding by her application during ADL tasks; ask about how she performs ADL tasks at home.
	4. Instruct in manipulation of clothing and bathing items while standing in walker at sink without violating hip precautions.

Functional Problem: ↓ dynamic balance during ADL tasks.

LTGs: By discharge (5/7/01) pt. will be Ⓘ and safe in toileting using adaptive equipment (walker and bedside commode).

STG	Interventions
1. Pt. Ⓘ in sit ↔ stand using walker in 2 tx sessions while observing total hip precautions.	1. Instruct pt. in safe transfer techniques; reinforce compliance with total hip precautions.
2. Pt. will transfer with SBA sit ↔ stand using bedside commode and manage clothing with no more than 2 verbal cues by next tx. session.	2. Provide UE strengthening through reaching and wt. bearing activities at sink and closet for grooming and dressing items and pushing up from chair and bedside commode.
3. Pt. will be assessed for possible continued home visits and home equipment procurement if progress warrants d/c to home by 3rd tx session.	3. Interview pt. regarding home environment; explore and discuss interim living arrangements or possible equipment use and placement in home; discuss support services needed if d/c to home is warranted.

Discharge Plan: To assisted living facility for 3 to 4 wks. until safe in completing all ADL tasks Ⓘ at home with assistance of home health aide if warranted by progress.

Treatment Plan: Cancer

Hospital and Rehabilitation Center Treatment Plan

Name: Carol M. **Age:** 35 **Primary Dx:** Ⓛ mastectomy 2° breast CA

Strengths: Prior to surgery Carol was in good physical condition and employed full time. She has some social support from her sister who lives in another state.

Functional Problem: Carol avoids social outings with friends due to ↓ self-esteem secondary to cosmetic alterations imposed by mastectomy procedure, which precludes her ability to return to work.

LTG: Carol will ↑ social interactions and activity to six outings/month within the next month, in preparation for return to work.

STG	Interventions
1. Carol will identify one support group of interest to her within 1 week in order to ↑ willingness to be out in public for work and social activities.	1. Educate Carol re: available support groups and peer visitation groups, their contact persons, telephone numbers, and ask her whether or not she has made contact.
2. Carol will attend 1 support group activity within 2 wks in order to ↑ confidence in social and work situations.	2. Accompany Carol into the community the first time she goes out.
3. Carol will initiate conversation with at least one other support member during her first visit to the group in order to ↓ negative impact of cosmetic alterations to body image.	3. Discuss Carol's experiences in the support groups with her.
4. Carol will enroll in a women's exercise program in order to ↑ activity tolerance and positive body image.	4. Educate Carol re: area exercise groups for post-mastectomy patients.
5. Carol will identify five assets she possesses other than physical in order to ↑ self-esteem and confidence in social and work situations.	5. Discuss Carol's assets with her, encouraging her to think of as many as she can.

Functional Problem: Carol is unable to return to work 2° 3/4 AROM, 4-/5 muscle strength, ↓ activity tolerance (fatigues after 1 hr.), and sensory changes.

LTG: Carol will return to work part time by 8/8/01.

STG	Interventions
1. Carol will demonstrate activity tolerance of 2 hours for work tasks within 3 weeks.	1. Scar massage and myofascial release to incision area along with pt. education on self-massage.
2. Carol will demonstrate ↑ of 20° in Ⓛ shoulder flexion in order to be able to reach the items she needs to work.	2. PROM to Ⓛ shoulder — instruct in self-ranging program.
3. Carol will demonstrate strength of 5- in Ⓛ shoulder musculature in order to be able to complete repetitive tasks at work.	3. Resistive strengthening with theratubing, weights, and graded functional activities. Active resistive ROM to Ⓛ UE.
4. Carol will use correct body mechanics in seated and active work tasks to have pain level of <2/10 while working.	4. Provide home exercise program and modify as patient progresses. Provide education on women's exercise groups.
5. Carol will observe sensory precautions in work and daily living tasks. Work simulation with patient education on energy conservation principles. Educate in ergonomics and posture in order to prevent pain.	5. Provide education on safety concerns with sensory loss.

Progress Note: Hand Therapy

Hand Therapy Clinic Progress Note

Date: 6/11/01 **Time:** 1:00 PM

S: Client reports pain @ the ulnar styloid with forearm supination. Client reports she is still unable to start her car c̄ her Ⓡ hand but can now use it to turn a doorknob.

O: Client seen in hand clinic for functional range of motion in Ⓡ UE. Moist heat applied to Ⓡ hand and forearm for 10 minutes prior to beginning treatment.

A/PROM Measurements for hand and forearm are:

[KEY: extension/flexion; ( ) PROM; - extension lag; + hyperextension]

Ⓡ hand	MP	PIP	DIP
Index	0/90	0/105	0/75
Long	0/90	0/105	0/80
Ring	0/90	0/105	0/80
Small	0/90	-14/105 (0/105)	0/79

Ⓡ wrist: +45/40 (+60/50) composite
Ⓡ forearm: Supination 62 (78) Pronation 90

Client performed the following exercises c̄ Ⓡ UE: Isometric forearm supination x10, AAROM supination x5, AROM forearm supination x5. After exercise, client's supination ↑ to 77° AROM. HEP revised to include blue foam for flexion strengthening 2 to 3x/day.

A: Client's gains in DIP flexion AROM since last week are due to ↑ strength of flexors. Active wrist flexion ↑ 9° and extension ↑ 5° from last week. ↑ in active pronation is due to ↑ strength while client lost 14° of forearm supination since last week which appears to be a result of muscle tightness. Client would benefit from continued skilled OT to regain FROM to complete IADLs and for general strengthening.

P: Client to be seen 2x/wk for 30-minute sessions. Continue wrist exercises and modify home exercise plan to include more supination stretching and strengthening. Client will demonstrate Ⓘ in HEP and sufficient ↑ in forearm supination to start her car c̄ Ⓡ UE in 2 weeks.

Progress Note: Mental Health

Behavioral Health Center Progress Note

Date: 5/21/02 Time: 4:00 pm

S: During the first 3 days of admission, Ms. Jones elected not to attend occupational therapy group sessions, maintaining that she was too "anxious and overwhelmed."

O: Client stayed in her room most of the time for first 3 days despite consistent invitations to attend groups. On this day the client attended a stress management group. Initially she was quiet, but gradually began entering into the activity. She was able to identify specific physical, emotional, and behavioral symptoms that she experiences when feeling overwhelmed or anxious. Ms. Jones stated that she had not been aware of these stress reactions.

A: The client is making progress as indicated by her initiating attendance to group, as well as relaxing and opening up socially during the group. Additional progress indicated by recognizing specific symptoms of stress as opposed to relating only general feelings.

P: Continue all goals as originally stated. Client to be seen daily to provide opportunities for Ms. Jones to learn basic stress management techniques so that she may recognize and control stress reactions when she begins feeling overwhelmed or anxious.

Discharge Note (SOAP format)

Hospital and Rehabilitation Center
Occupational Therapy Discharge Summary

Patient: Ted
OT order received: 2/7/02
Number of treatments: 5
Admit Date: 1/29/02
OT Evaluation completed: 2/8/02
Discharge Date: 2/16/02

S: Pt. reports "doing a lot better" and being "less confused" than he was on admission.

O: Pt. initially presented with head trauma 2° to MVA. Occupational therapy evaluation on 2/8/02 indicated pt. had deficits in short-term memory, safety awareness, attention to task, and ADL status. Pt. seen 30 minutes daily for 5 days for ADL retraining for dressing, grooming, and functional mobility. Pt. and family received skilled instruction in safety precautions in the home. Pt.'s functional status on admit and discharge as follows:

Goal #	Admit status	Goal	D/C status
1	Min Ⓐ in grooming	Set-up/supervision	Set-up/supervision
2	CGA in toilet transfers	SBA	SBA
3	Supine ↔ sit with min Ⓐ	SBA	SBA
4	Min Ⓐ UE dressing	Set-up/supervision	Set-up/supervision

A: All goals achieved due to improved cognitive status, awareness of safety precautions, and skilled instruction in ADLs. Pt. will need supervision at home 2° remaining cognitive (attention and short-term memory) deficits.

P: Pt. discharged to home. Recommend home health occupational therapy evaluation for safety in home environment and potential for necessary durable medical equipment. No home exercise program given. No other referrals at time of discharge. OT will follow up in 1 month by phone to check pt.'s functional status in the home.

Discharge Note (Facility format)

Hospital and Rehabilitation Center Discharge Summary

Name: Marjorie Patient
Physician: Fred Dietrich, MD
Start of Care: 4/1/02
Primary Dx: CVA
Medical Record#: 97865
Room #: 537
Date of Discharge: 4/10/02
Secondary Dx: Arthritis

_X_ Occupational Therapy ____ Physical Therapy ____ Communicative Disorders

Course of Treatment: Client seen daily for 9 days, 30 minutes each session following CVA to work on ↑ independence in self-care skills, functional mobility, UE strengthening, energy conservation, and activity tolerance.

Status on Discharge: Client reports feeling much better and is ready to go home.

Discharge Status	Admit Status
Self-care Ⓘ and safe	Self-care mod Ⓐ
Functional mobility Ⓘ and safe	Functional mobility mod Ⓐ
Activity tolerance 8 minutes for ADL tasks	Activity tolerance 10 minutes for ADL tasks

Goals Met: Client has met self-care and functional mobility goals using energy conservation techniques.

Goals Not Met: Activity tolerance goal not met due to client refusing last two treatment sessions when she learned she was being discharged.

Patient/Family Education: Client instructed in and demonstrates understanding of HEP. Handouts given. Client reports having weights at home she can use for continued UE strengthening as instructed in her HEP.

Recommendations: Discharge client to her sister's home due to goals being met. HEP attached. No home health recommended at this time.

The notes that follow are examples of SOAP notes that could be written by an OTA in a variety of work settings. While we cannot represent each and every unique setting in which an OTA may work, we hope to provide you with a small sampling of this form of documentation.

Treatment Note: Acute Care

Hospital and Rehabilitation Center Acute Care Unit
Occupational Therapy Treatment Note

Date: 4/22/02 **Time:** 3:00 pm

S: Pt. nonverbal. Pt. demonstrated startle response c̄ position change.

O: Pt. seen bedside to work on initiating and attending to self-care task. When asked to point finger, pt. required multiple verbal cues and demonstrations, and demonstrated poor response time. Pt. requires max Ⓐ supine → sit EOB. Pt. required multiple verbal cues and hand over hand Ⓐ 75% of the time to initiate holding on to washcloth. Pt. able to place washcloth in water with one verbal cue but required hand over hand Ⓐ to bring washcloth to face. Pt. attended to looking at self in mirror for ~1 minute. Pt. required hand over hand Ⓐ to initiate brushing hair. Shoulder AROM limited due to ↓ tone.

A: Overall, pt.'s motor planning, task initiation, and attention during treatment activities continue to be limited. Pt. would benefit from ranging activities to increase shoulder elevation, as well as further interventions focusing on the skills of initiating and attending to task in order to complete ADL activities.

P: Pt. to continue occupational therapy daily for 20-minute sessions until discharge in ~4 weeks to work on self-care activities and the underlying performance components necessary to complete tasks Ⓘ. Pt. will follow a 1-step command in 1 week in order to attend to self-care routine.

Treatment Note: Cognition

Hospital Occupational Therapy Treatment Note

Date: 4/5/02 Time: 10:00 AM

S: Veteran reports feeling fine, but says he does not remember the OTA's name that he has been working with.

O: Veteran seen in occupational therapy clinic for cognitive tasks, Ⓡ UE AROM, strengthening, and fine motor coordination. Veteran oriented to person, month, year, and place after prompting. He followed 2-step commands after max verbal cues and mod physical assist to complete basic self-care tasks. Veteran was unable to grasp and release items with Ⓡ hand. He required mod physical and verbal cues to complete UE AROM used in table top activities.

A: Veteran is not oriented to surroundings at all times, which presents safety concerns. His ↓ cognitive functioning leads to ↓ attention to completion of tasks, specifically dressing, feeding, and bathing. Veteran would benefit from cognitive skills training and safety instruction. Veteran also displays ↓ strength, coordination, and AROM in Ⓡ UE that limits his ability to complete ADL activities. He would benefit from instruction in using Ⓡ UE as an assist as well as from activities to ↑ Ⓡ UE strength, AROM, and coordination to perform self-care activities.

P: Veteran will continue to receive treatment daily for 4 weeks for 1 hour to improve cognitive skills, ↑ attention to task and safety awareness, and to ↑ Ⓡ UE strength, AROM, and coordination in order to complete self-care tasks. Veteran will attend to task for 3 minutes in order to complete morning grooming within 2 weeks.

Treatment Note: Home Health Mental Health

Community Support Services Contact Note

Name: John Williams **Date:** 2/14/02 **Beginning Time:** 9:00 AM **Ending Time:** 10:15 AM
Length of Service: 75 minutes **Goals:** 2, 4, and 5

S: John states that having a bank account instead of keeping all his money in cash in an envelope is very confusing to him, and he is never sure anymore how much money he has. He also reported some continuing confusion regarding his medication.

O: John was seen in his home to fill his mediset and review his grocery needs. Skilled instruction provided in meal planning and calculating probable food costs. He was then taken to the bank to withdraw some money, and to a local grocery store to purchase food. At the bank, the teller figured John's account, which confused him. Skilled instruction provided in calculating a bank balance. At the grocery store, purchased canned fruits and vegetables, ground beef, fresh lettuce, and a loaf of bread. Upon returning home he put the lettuce and meat in the refrigerator Ⓘ and consulted his weekly menu planner to determine what he had planned for lunch.

A: John needed only two verbal cues to fill his mediset with correct doses of all medications this week as opposed to four verbal cues last week. Understanding a bank balance is a new skill for John and he needs continued skilled instruction and opportunities to apply his new knowledge before he is able to manage the account Ⓘ. He continues to make progress in choosing healthy foods as evidenced by his choice of canned fruits and vegetables and the addition of lettuce to his sandwiches. John could benefit from continued skilled instruction in ADL skills such as Ⓘ management of medication, food, and money in order to be able to live Ⓘ in the community without the support of a professional staff.

P: John will continue to be seen weekly in his home and community settings in order to work toward Ⓘ in meeting his daily needs. John will fill his mediset Ⓘ without verbal cues within 3 weeks in order to ↓ the amount of support needed to comply with his medication regimen.

TREATMENT NOTE: MENTAL HEALTH

MENTAL HEALTH CENTER OCCUPATIONAL THERAPY TREATMENT NOTE

Date: 4/16/02 **Time:** 4:00 pm

S: Client reported she is currently not volunteering and has not worked for the past 4 years due to her disability status. Regarding volunteering, she says, "I need the structure," and further stated that she wants to be productive. Currently, client reports she sleeps "too much," and is having relationship problems.

O: Client was admitted yesterday and attended 4/4 group sessions today. During expressive therapy group, client participated in baking with the rest of the group, but did not eat anything. When each group member identified current emotions, client identified hers as miserable, angry, very anxious, over-stimulated, frustrated, frightened, and alienated. During ADL skills group, client identified a possible problem she may encounter upon discharge to be lack of organization, with her "red flags" being over-sleeping and agitation. Client welcomed suggestions from others regarding structuring her time.

A: Client is very perceptive of her emotions and limitations. Her refusal to eat with the group indicates continued appetite disturbance. Client would benefit from information about eating disorders. She would also benefit from continued group participation, with emphasis on increasing self-esteem and time management skills. Client's participation in all four group sessions today indicates good rehab potential.

P: Client will continue to attend all daily group sessions while on the acute unit to work on increasing self-esteem and ability to structure her time. Client will demonstrate increased time management skills by naming five strategies she will use for gaining control of her daily time by D/C in approximately 4 days.

TREATMENT NOTE: PEDIATRIC (PRESCHOOL AGE)

CHILDREN'S CENTER OCCUPATIONAL THERAPY TREATMENT NOTE

Date: 4/7/02 Time: 3:00 PM

S: Mary said she wanted to play, but when the task was difficult for her, she said, "You do it. You fix it."

O: Mary seen for 45 minutes in her home to work on Ⓑ use of UE to ↑ spontaneous use of Ⓛ hand as a functional assist, sitting balance while tailor sitting unsupported, and functional mobility, as a prerequisite to self-care and play skills. Mary was engaged during ~90% of the session.

Bilateral UE Use: Mary required max Ⓐ to pull shirt over stuffed animal's arms with Ⓡ UE while holding it with Ⓛ UE. She spontaneously used Ⓛ hand to assist with stabilizing animal while pulling sleeve over its arm and shoulder c̄ hand. Mary initiated snapping shirt, but needed max Ⓐ to use Ⓛ hand to stabilize shirt while fastening snaps. Ⓑ hands used to hold animal steady during play.

Sitting Balance: Mary requires touch cues from stand → sit in walker and mod physical Ⓐ from side sit → cross-legged sit. She demonstrated adequate sitting balance to play for 5 minutes, requiring tactile cues twice to right herself from a lateral tilt.

A: Mary demonstrated Ⓑ coordination and use of Ⓛ hand as a functional assist ~60% of the time, which is an increase from last week. When she is engrossed in activity, Mary is unable to concentrate on postural support, and needs CGA assist to resume upright posture. She would benefit from continued skilled OT for activities which challenge postural support in order to gain protective responses, body righting, and vestibular integration in order to ↑ her Ⓘ during play.

P: Mary will continue to be seen 45 minutes once a week for next 7 weeks to continue strengthening postural support in order to ↑ her Ⓘ in play activities and promote Ⓑ hand use and ↑ use of the Ⓛ hand as a functional assist during ADL and play activities. Mary will be able to maintain upright posture for 10 minutes without lateral tilt within 3 weeks.

Treatment Note: Public School

Children's Center Visit Note

Date: 4/12/01 **Time:** 2:30 pm

S: Heather did not use verbal language to communicate, but did echo words spoken to her.

O: Heather was seen in classroom to work on fine motor skills to prepare for scissors and improve prehension patterns for writing. After 5 minutes of brushing to decrease tactile sensitivity, Heather worked on palmar pinch and tripod grasp prehension patterns using a cereal bracelet activity for 20 minutes. Heather used tongs (in preparation for scissors use) to pull 15 circle-shaped pieces of cereal out of a cup one at a time. Then using a palmar pinch, she placed each piece of cereal over a pipe cleaner. Five verbal cues were required for task completion.

A: Heather manipulates tongs well and exhibits a good awareness of positioning of tongs within her hands, which is an indicator that proper scissors use will be attained soon. Good attention to task for entire 25 minutes shows good potential to meet stated goals.

P: Continue prehension activities 3 x/wk. using a variety of media in 20- to 30-minute intervals until proper scissors use goal is achieved. Heather will be able to cut a piece of 8"x10" paper ~ in half using adaptive spring scissors Ⓘ by 2/19/02.

Treatment Note: Prosthetic Adaptation

Hospital and Rehabilitation Center
Occupational Therapy Note

Name: Daniel Patient **Date:** 2/5/02 **Time:** 3:06 PM **Physician:** Dr. Woodard
Medical Record #: 87654 **Room #:** 455W

S: Pt. appeared pleased with adaptations to prosthetic leg fasteners made this date stating, "This will work."

O: Pt. seen in rehab gym for adaptations necessary to don/doff prosthesis. Pt. sit ↔ stand Ⓘ from w/c while keeping one hand on walker for support. Pt. positioned prosthetic leg and attempted to fasten straps. Pt. mod Ⓐ in fastening of straps, Ⓘ in undoing of straps to doff prosthesis. Adaptations of prosthetic leg harness completed this date.

A: Inability to don prosthesis Ⓘ currently limits Ⓘ with ambulation/functional toileting. Pt. would benefit from additional skilled instruction in use of pulley-like fasteners on prosthesis to allow one-handed closure installed this date.

P: Continue skilled occupational therapy treatment for 2 more days to modify closing device on prosthesis and provide instruction and training in its use. Pt. will don/doff prosthesis Ⓘ with added pulley system using strap/loop/velcro by end of next tx session.

Treatment Note: Splint

Hospital and Treatment Center Outpatient Clinic
Occupational Therapy Note

Date: 1/21/01 **Time:** 3:00 PM

S: Mr. J. stated that the pain in his right wrist and thumb was "not as bad as it was 2 weeks ago." He reported that his splint is rubbing a calcium deposit on the dorsum of his hand and that he is not wearing the splint at work during the day. He also reported feeling pain during treatment with movement of the Ⓡ thumb, and that ice and iontopheresis ↓ pain.

O: Mr. J. arrived at clinic wearing forearm based thumb spica splint. Upon removal of splint, wrist appeared slightly swollen.

AROM: wrist flexion ~25%, wrist extension <25%, thumb MP flexion and extension ~25%

Mr. J. tolerated ~3 minutes friction massage over abductor pollicis longus and extensor pollicis brevis tendons. Ice applied for 5 minutes; Mr. J. instructed in using ice at home and at work to ↓ pain by ↓ inflammation of tendons. Splint reformed to eliminate rubbing on dorsum of hand, and Mr. J. instructed in a wearing schedule to use at work. HEP modified and Mr. J. demonstrated new procedures correctly.

A: Swelling ↓ since last tx. session. Wrist and thumb AROM are ~50% below functional limits, due to pain upon movement. Limited AROM & pain are causing functional problems in the work environment. Ice and iontopheresis ↓ pain and therefore ↑ functional ability c̄ Ⓡ hand. Splint reconstruction will also contribute to ↓ pain. Mr. J. would benefit from continued skilled OT to ↓ pain, ↑ AROM, ↑ ability to use hand at work.

P: Continue to see Mr. J. 2x/wk for the following:

- Ice & iontopheresis to ↓ pain in Ⓡ hand and wrist.
- Friction massage to ↓ inflammation and ↑ AROM in Ⓡ wrist and thumb.
- Reevaluation of splint for fit and use after reconstruction.
- Reevaluation of effectiveness and compliance of HEP.
- To achieve goal of ↓ pain in Ⓡ wrist and hand for use in functional activity at work and home, pt. will use a screwdriver during work task for 3 min. with <3/10 on pain scale within 2 visits (1 wk).

Bibliography

Abdelhak, M., Grostick, S., Hanken, M. A., & Jacobs, E. (Eds.). (1996). *Health information: Management of a strategic resource*. Philadelphia: W. B. Saunders.

Accreditation Council for Occupational Therapy Education. (1999). Standards for an accredited educational program for the occupational therapy assistant. *Am J Occup Ther, 53*(6),583-589.

American Occupational Therapy Association. (2000). Occupational therapy code of ethics (2000). *Am J Occup Ther, 54*(6), 614-616.

American Occupational Therapy Association. (1998). Standards of practice for occupational therapy. *Am J Occup Ther, 52*(10), 866-869.

American Occupational Therapy Association. (1995). Concept paper: Service delivery in occupational therapy. *Am J Occup Ther, 49*(10), 1029-1031.

American Occupational Therapy Association Intercommission Council. (1993). Occupational therapy roles. *Am J Occup Ther, 47*(12), 1087-1099.

American Occupational Therapy Association Managed Care Project Team. (1996). *Managed care: An occupational therapy sourcebook*. Bethesda, MD: American Occupational Therapy Association.

American Occupational Therapy Association Terminology Task Force. (1994). Uniform Terminology for occupational therapy—third edition. *Am J Occup Ther, 48*(11),1047-1054.

Backhaus, H., & Sladyk, K. (2001). Documentation. In K. Sladyk and S. Ryan (Eds.), *Ryan's occupational therapy assistant: Principles, practice issues, and techniques*. (3rd ed., pp. 403-411). Thorofare, NJ: SLACK Incorporated.

Cullen, C. (1998). *Physical disabilities and geriatric treatment plans: Medicare documentation for therapy services*. Retrieved from http://www.geocities.com/Heartland/Prairies/5309/

Fowler, R. (2001, February 19). Capitol briefing: Are you following your state's supervision regulations? *OT Practice Online*. Retrieved from http://www.aoto.org/featured/area2/

Hirama, H. (1996). *Occupational therapy assistant: A primer*. Baltimore: CHESS.

Huffman, E. K., & Cofer, J. (1994). *Health information management* (10th ed.). Berwyn, IL: Physician's Record.

Kannenberg, K. (1998). Special consideration III: Mental health. In J. D. Acquaviva (Ed.), *Effective documentation for occupational therapy* (2nd ed., pp. 115-129). Bethesda, MD: American Occupational Therapy Association.

Lopes, M. (1998). *Medicare guidelines explained for the occupational therapist*. Gaylord, MI: Northern Speech Services.

Mason, K. (2001). *Dyadic and group dynamics: Psychosocial SOAP notes*. Unpublished manuscript.

Moyers, P. A. (1999). *The guide to occupational therapy practice* [special issue]. *Am J Occup Ther, 53*(3).

O'Hara, D. J. (1990). *Guidelines for SOAP notes*. Unpublished manuscript. University of Missouri-Columbia.

Pedretti, L. W. (1996). *Occupational therapy: Practice skills for physical dysfunction* (4th ed.). St. Louis, MO: Mosby.

Perinchief, J. M. (1998). Management of occupational therapy. In M. E. Neistadt & E. B. Crepeau (Eds.), *Willard and Spackman's occupational therapy* (9th ed., pp. 772-790). Philadelphia: Lippincott, Williams, & Wilkins.

Pinson, C. (1998). Documentation review. In J. D. Acquaviva (Ed.), *Effective documentation for occupational therapy* (2nd ed., pp. 149-206). Bethesda, MD: American Occupational Therapy Association.

Ramsey, R. M., & Auerbach, E. (1997). Forms follow function: Documentation for reimbursement in mental health OT. *OT Practice, 2*, 20-23.

Thomson, L. K., & Foto, M. (1995). Elements of clinical documentation (revision). *Am J Occup Ther, 49*(10), 1031-1035.

Suggestions for Completing the Worksheets

The worksheets in this manual were originally developed for use as in-class exercises. In a classroom situation, students are asked to collaborate on an answer and their collaborative efforts are recorded on a flip chart or blackboard. This is a particularly nonthreatening way for students to learn new skills, since it allows them to try out ideas and hear the ideas of others as they work toward a correct result. In this situation, the instructor can guide their efforts by asking questions to facilitate good clinical reasoning.

In our experience, many of these exercises do not work as well when used as homework assignments. Because there are so many "correct" ways to complete them, they can be grading nightmares. The suggestions offered here as "good" or "correct" are only a few of the many possible correct answers. As you do the exercises with a class, you may collect many more equally "good" answers.

If you are a new therapist or a student using this manual, rather than an instructor, you should be able to work your way through the exercises and check your work against those in this Appendix. Remember that your answer can be different and still be correct, as long as it contains the essential elements. You should not sacrifice your own writing style to be more like someone else's, as long as your information and protocol are essentially correct.

SOAP notes are very difficult to write if there is no treatment session about which to write. Although there are many examples in this manual, there is no substitute for observing or working with actual patients. Only then will you be able to translate your treatment session onto paper in a meaningful way.

CHAPTER 2

Worksheet 2-1: Using Abbreviations

Translate each sentence written with abbreviations into full English phrases or sentences using Table 2-1.

- Pt. c/o pain in Ⓡ MCP joint p̄ ~15 min. PROM.

  Patient complained of pain in the right metacarpophalangeal joint after approximately 15 minutes of passive range of motion.

- Pt. w/c → mat c̄ sliding board max Ⓐ x2.

  Patient transferred from his wheelchair to the mat using a sliding board and maximum assistance of two people.

- Pt. O x4.

  The patient was oriented to person, time, place, and situation.

- Pt. able to don pants SBA c̄ verbal cues to thread Ⓛ LE.

  The patient was able to put on his pants with stand-by assistance, but needed verbal cues to be able to thread his left foot into the leg hole.

- 1° dx. THR 2° dx. COPD & CHF.

  Primary diagnosis is total hip replacement. Secondary diagnoses are chronic obstructive pulmonary disease and congestive heart failure.

Shorten these notes using only the standard abbreviations in this chapter.

- Patient has thirty degrees of passive range of motion in the left distal interphalangeal joint, which is within functional limits.

  30° PROM in Ⓛ DIP is WFL.

- Patient is able to put on her socks with standby assistance, but requires moderate assistance with putting on and taking off left shoe.

  Pt. dons socks SBA but requires mod Ⓐ to don & doff Ⓛ shoe.

- The patient requires contact guard assistance for balance during her morning dressing, which she performs while sitting on the edge of her bed.

  CGA *for balance for* AM *dressing* EOB.

Worksheet 2-2: Additional Practice

Shorten these notes using the standard abbreviations in Table 2-1.

- The patient was seen bedside for training in activities of daily living. She was able to perform bed mobility exercises with moderate assistance, but needed maximum assistance to put on her Depends. She was able to go from a supine position to a sitting position with minimum assistance and from a sitting position to a standing position with moderate assistance.

  Pt. seen bedside for ADL training. Mod Ⓐ bed mobility, max Ⓐ to don Depends. Supine → sit min Ⓐ and sit → stand mod Ⓐ.

- The resident came to the occupational therapy clinic via wheelchair escort. The resident was observed to lean to his left. The resident needed verbal cues and minimum assistance in positioning his body in the wheelchair to maintain midline orientation and symmetrical posture. The resident transferred from his wheelchair to the toilet with moderate assistance of one person using a standing pivot transfer. He needed verbal cues and visual feedback from a mirror to maintain upright posture.

  Resident to OT via w/c escort. Resident leans Ⓛ and needs verbal cues and min. physical Ⓐ to maintain symmetrical posture in midline. Standing pivot transfer w/c → toilet mod Ⓐ. Verbal cues and feedback using a mirror needed to maintain upright posture.

- The veteran has been treated three out of five times in the past week. Two treatments were missed due to urinary tract infection. The veteran's short-term memory was three out of three for immediate recall, one out of three after one minute, and zero out of three with verbal cues after five minutes. The left upper extremity shoulder flexion was a grade of four, shoulder extension was a grade of four, elbow flexion was a grade of four, elbow extension was a grade of four, wrist extension was a grade of three minus, wrist flexion was a grade of three minus, and grip strength was at eight pounds. The right upper extremity muscle grades are within normal limits.

  Veteran has been treated in OT 3/5 times in past week. 2 txs were missed 2° UTI. Short-term memory 3/3 immediate recall, 1/3 p̄ 1 minute, 0/3 c̄ verbal cues p̄ 5 min. Ⓛ UE shoulder and elbow strength grade 4, Ⓛ wrist strength grade 3-, grip strength 8#, Ⓡ UE all WNL.

- The patient is a sixty-three year old female who had coronary artery bypass graft surgery. Her past medical history includes diabetes mellitus type 2, hypertension, coronary artery disease, and degenerative joint disease. Her date of discharge from the skilled nursing home was April 1, 2000.

  Pt. is 63 y.o. ♀ s/p CABG. *Hx includes* DM *type 2,* HTN, CAD, DJD. *D/C from* SNF *4/01/2000.*

CHAPTER 3

Worksheet 3-1: Writing Concise, Coherent Statements

During a treatment session your patient makes the following statements:

- "I used that dressing stick and sock aide like you showed me to get dressed without bending down this morning."
- "My hip doesn't hurt when I stand up or sit down, especially with that new toilet seat you got for me."
- "It's getting easier for me to get dressed now."

- "My daughter said they delivered all that bathroom equipment to her house yesterday."

Using these statements, write your own concise and organized version for the "S" portion of the SOAP note.

Pt. reports using adaptive equipment to don pants and socks while maintaining hip precautions without difficulty. She has no c/o pain with transfers using raised toilet seat. Her daughter now has bathroom equipment in home that was ordered by OT last week.

Worksheet 3-2: Choosing a Subjective Statement

Which would be best to use as the subjective section of the SOAP note?

1. Even though the patient may have been cooperative, and even though it may have been important in this treatment session, it is an assessment of the situation, and does not belong in the "S" category of the note. The patient's social conversation might be important in some situations. However, there is a better choice for this particular note.
2. In this instance, a pending visit by the patient's grandson is not really relevant to the treatment session or to how the patient sees her progress. It might be important in another situation. For example, if the patient were planning to go to live with her grandson after discharge, it might be very relevant, and might be a topic the OTA wanted to explore further with the patient.
3. Feeling "pretty good" today might be important, because it might show progress or a change in her condition. In this case, however, it is not the best choice.
4. ***The patient's observations about her upper extremity seem most pertinent to this treatment session. Use of the Ⓡ UE is relevant in all aspects of this treatment session.***
5. A report of safety concerns by nursing might be relevant to this patient's treatment. However, it is not the best choice for the "S" category of this note, for several reasons. A concern by nursing staff should be documented in the nursing notes. The OTA should report what she sees, rather than what some other staff member believes. Finally, the subjective section of the SOAP note is used to document the patient's views about treatment rather than the staff's views, except in rare instances.

Chapter 4

Worksheet 4-1: Choosing Categories

How would you divide this information into categores to make it easier to read?

- *Ⓛ UE use*
- *Feeding*
- *Attention to task or attention span*
- *Splint*

Worksheet 4-2: Being Specific About Assist Levels

Rewrite the statements below to provide a part of the task that required assistance. Since you have not seen the patient, you cannot know what really required assistance.

1. Pt. supine → sit with min Ⓐ, bed → w/c with mod Ⓐ.
   - Pt. supine → sit with min Ⓐ, bed → w/c with mod Ⓐ for balance.
   - Pt. supine → sit with min Ⓐ, bed → w/c with mod Ⓐ to lift body weight.
   - Pt. supine → sit with min Ⓐ, bed → w/c with mod Ⓐ to bring hips and trunk to 45°.
   - Pt. supine → sit with min Ⓐ swinging legs to EOB, bed → w/c with mod Ⓐ for postural control.
2. Pt. required SBA in transferring w/c → toilet
   - Pt. required SBA in transferring w/c → toilet for proper hand placement.
   - Pt. required SBA in transferring w/c → toilet to push up with arms from wheelchair.
   - Pt. required SBA in transferring w/c → toilet to remind him of steps of the transfer.

3. Pt. retrieved garments from low drawers with min Ⓐ.
   - Pt. retrieved garments from low drawers with min Ⓐ to open drawers.
   - Pt. retrieved garments from low drawers with min Ⓐ to release trigger on reacher.
   - Pt. retrieved garments from low drawers with min Ⓐ to judge halo placement in space.
   - Pt. retrieved garments from low drawers with min Ⓐ to grasp handles of drawers.
4. Brushing hair required max Ⓐ.
   - Brushing hair required max Ⓐ to reach back of head.
   - Brushing hair required max Ⓐ to flex shoulder past 35°.
5. Pt. completed dressing, toileting, and hygiene with min Ⓐ.
   - Pt. completed dressing, toileting, and hygiene with min Ⓐ to reach feet.
   - Pt. completed dressing, toileting, and hygiene with min Ⓐ for activities requiring fine motor dexterity.
   - Pt. completed dressing, toileting, and hygiene with min Ⓐ to adhere to hip precautions.

Worksheet 4-3: De-Emphasizing the Treatment Media

Rewrite the following statements to emphasize the skilled occupational therapy that is actually occuring in the treatment session:

1. Patient played pegboard game to work on functional grasp.

   Patient worked on functional grasp/release patterns needed to handle small objects for grooming and dressing.
2. Patient played catch using bilateral UEs to facilitate grasp and release pattern.

   Pt. worked on functional grasp/release patterns needed to manipulate household objects.
3. Patient put dirt into pot to ½-way point, added seedling, and filled remainder of pot with dirt transferred by cup. Pt. completed 3 more pots while standing 8 minutes before requiring a 5-minute rest. Pt. resumed standing position to water completed pots for approximately 5 minutes.

   Pt. demonstrated standing tolerance of 13 minutes with a 5-minute break after 8 minutes in order to prepare for standing to complete ADL tasks.

Worksheet 4-4: Being Concise

Reword the following note to be more concise:

O: Pt. seen bedside. Pt. ambulated ~36 inches to shower with SBA. Pt. instructed to complete shower while sitting. Pt. performed shower with SBA to manage IV line. Pt. able to wash upper and lower body Ⓘ and dry entire body after completing shower. Pt. required ~20 minutes to complete shower. Pt. then ambulated ~36 inches to chair and sat. Pt. needed verbal cues to remain seated while donning underwear and pants. Pt. able to dress UE Ⓘ and lower body p̄ verbal cues for sitting. Pt. demonstrated good sitting balance, but needed SBA for standing. Following shower, pt. stated he would like to take a nap and was assisted back into bed.

Pt. seen in room for skilled instruction in self-care activities. Ambulated ~3 ft. to and from shower c̄ SBA to manage IV line while ambulating and showering. Shower took ~20 minutes. Pt. showered and dressed p̄ verbal cues to sit. Pt. demonstrated good sitting balance but required SBA for balance while standing. Following shower, pt. assisted back into bed.

- OR -

Pt. seen in room for skilled instruction in safe showering and dressing. Pt. ambulated ~3' SBA for balance. After verbal cues to sit, pt. showered in 20 min c̄ SBA to manage IV lines. Dressed UE Ⓘ while seated and LE c̄ verbal cues to remain seated.

Chapter 5

Worksheet 5-1: Justifying Continued Treatment

Which of the following require the skill of an OTA?

No The practice of coordination and self-care skills on a daily basis.

Yes Modifying functional tasks/activities through the provision of adaptive equipment or techniques.

Yes Determining that the modified task is safe and effective.

No Carrying out a maintenance program.
Yes Teaching the patient to use the breathing techniques he has been taught while performing his ADL activities.
Yes Providing individualized instruction to the patient, family, or caregiver.
Yes Provision of specialized instruction to eliminate limitations in a functional activity.
Yes Instructing caregivers.
Yes Making changes in the environment.
Yes Teaching compensatory skills.
No Gait training.
Yes Intervening with patients to eliminate safety hazards.
No Presenting information handouts (such as energy conservation) without having the patient perform the activity.
No Routine exercise and strengthening programs.
Yes Adding instruction in lower body dressing techniques to a current ADL program.
Yes Teaching adaptive techniques such as one-handed shoe tying.
Yes Advancing a treatment plan that is in place.

Worksheet 5-2: Assessing the "Categories" Note

Write your assessment based on the information given [on the worksheet].

A: Safety concerns (impulsivity ↓ dynamic standing balance) noted when patient attempts to transfer sit → stand during toileting. Pt. verbalized an understanding of safety instructions and has potential to progress to independence. Pt.'s ↓ AROM in right shoulder, ↓ activity tolerance, and ↓ dynamic standing balance all interfere with ability to complete ADL tasks safely and independently. Pt. would benefit from Ⓡ UE AROM and strengthening exercises along with continued skilled instruction in safety issues and energy conservation techniques.

Worksheet 5-3: Assessing Problems Not Within Functional Limits

Rewrite the following statements using the formula given [on the worksheet].

Patient demonstrated difficulty with laundry and cooking tasks due to memory and sequencing deficits.
Memory and sequencing deficits cause difficulty c̄ home management tasks.

Decreased level of arousal noted during morning dressing activities, requiring redirection to task.
↓ level of arousal limits patient's ability to complete basic ADL tasks.

Patient unable to follow hip precautions during morning dressing due to memory deficits.
Memory deficits interfere c̄ patient's ability to incorporate hip precautions into basic self-care tasks.
-OR-
Memory deficits limit pt.'s ability to follow hip precautions while dressing.

Patient problem-solved poorly while performing lower body dressing as evidenced by multiple attempts to button pants and don socks.
Patient's ↓ ability to problem-solve limits her ability to dress herself s̄ Ⓐ and raises safety concerns in all ADL areas.

Worksheet 5-4: Assessing a Note

For any problem you identify, note the performance area that is affected.

Problems or Progress

The problems that stood out for this therapist as she wrote her note included:

- Trunk stability
- Asymmetrical posture
- Ⓛ UE AROM
- Decreased muscle strength

She decided that the problems with bilateral integration and inability to cross midline were a function of the decreased range and strength, rather than separate problems.

Rehab Potential

- Ability to follow directions/intact cognitive status
- Intact visual perceptual skills

She grouped the trunk stability and asymmetrical posture together, since in her professional judgment one was causing the other, and they constituted a safety problem in functional mobility. She grouped the UE AROM with the decreased muscle strength, which she felt to be causing abnormal reach patterns that interfered with transfers and with all self-care tasks.

Next, write an assessment of the observation based on the items you have listed.

Decreased trunk stability causes asymmetrical posture, which results in safety concerns during transfers. Decreased AROM in the Ⓛ UE results in decreased bilateral integration and midline crossing which decreases the patient's ability to perform basic ADL tasks. Ability to follow directions 100% of the time and good visual perceptual skills indicate good rehab potential. Patient would benefit from continued activities to increase trunk stability and AROM of the Ⓛ UE needed for dressing and transfers.

-OR-

A: Pt.'s ability to follow directions during treatment, ability to appropriately utilize visual/perceptual skills, and ability to follow verbal commands indicate good rehab potential. Pt.'s reduced AROM of Ⓛ UE and asymmetrical trunk posture currently limit Ⓘ and safe performance of transfers and ADL tasks. Pt. would benefit from skilled instruction of bilateral integration techniques in order to incorporate UE in self-care activities, as well as Ⓛ UE exercises to strengthen and↑ tone of Ⓛ UE in order to perform transfers and ADLs Ⓘ. Pt. would also benefit from skilled instruction in weight shifting techniques in order to improve trunk stability.

-OR-

A: Pt.'s intact cognitive status and ability to follow verbal commands indicate good rehab potential. Problems include decreased AROM and strength in Ⓛ UE and unstable trunk balance which limit Ⓘ in ADLs. Pt. would benefit from skilled OT to provide activities that increase AROM and strength in the Ⓛ UE, Brunnstrom balance exercises, and skilled instruction in safe transfers and dressing.

-OR-

A: Safety concerns with balance noted due to asymmetry of pt.'s trunk and shoulders. ↓ AROM of Ⓛ UE and difficulty with midline crossing interferes with ability to complete ADLs. Pt.'s ability to follow verbal commands indicates good rehab potential. Pt. would benefit from AROM and strengthening activities to improve posture, balance, and trunk stability. Pt. would also benefit from future midline crossing and Ⓑ activities to prepare for future ADL training.

CHAPTER 6

Worksheet 6-1: Final SOAP Note for a Treatment Session Written in "Categories"

Write your plan for this patient below:

P: Patient will continue to be treated 5 x/wk for 1 week for skilled instruction in safe transfers and toileting. Home program for AROM and strengthening exercises for Ⓡ shoulder will be taught. Pt. will demonstrate ability to transfer to toilet safely with CGA and use of walker and grab bars by the end of 5 tx sessions.

(Note by Tara Grantham)

Worksheet 6-2: Completing the Plan for the Postural Instability Note

Write your plan for this patient below:

P: Continue to treat pt. in OT 1 hour daily for 3 weeks to increase trunk stability. Within 1 week, patient will be able to sit EOB unsupported for >2 minutes in order to begin instruction in compensatory dressing techniques EOB next week.

Additional answers for Worksheet 6-2

Another therapist might have written the assessment and plan in a different way. Below are other possible assessments for this note, along with a plan for each.

A: Pt.'s ability to follow directions during treatment, ability to appropriately utilize visual/perceptual skills, and ability to follow verbal commands indicate good rehab potential. Pt.'s reduced AROM of Ⓛ UE and asymmetrical trunk posture currently limit Ⓘ and safe performance of transfers and ADL tasks. Pt. would benefit from skilled instruction of bilateral integration techniques in order to incorporate UE in self-care activities, as well as Ⓛ UE exercises to strengthen and ↑ tone of Ⓛ UE in order to perform transfers and ADLs Ⓘ . Pt. would also benefit from skilled instruction in weight shifting techniques in order to improve trunk stability.

P: Continue to treat pt. b.i.d. for 1 week in order to ↑ trunk stability, improve weight shifts, ↑ AROM of Ⓛ UE, and improve safety of transfers and ADLs. Pt. will demonstrate Ⓘ in ADL tasks by discharge on 1/7/02.

- OR-

A: Pt.'s intact cognitive status and ability to follow verbal commands indicate good rehab potential. Problems include ↓ AROM and strength in Ⓛ UE and unstable trunk balance which limit Ⓘ in ADLs. Pt. would benefit from skilled OT to provide activities that increase AROM and strength in the Ⓛ UE, Brunnstrom balance exercises and skilled instruction in safe transfers and dressing.

P: Continue to treat pt. b.i.d. for 1 week for Brunnstrom balance exercises in order to begin transfer training by 1/30/02.

- OR-

A: Safety concerns with balance noted due to asymmetry of pt.'s trunk and shoulders. ↓ AROM of Ⓛ UE and difficulty with midline crossing interferes with ability to complete ADLs. Pt.'s ability to follow verbal commands indicates good rehab potential. Pt. would benefit from AROM and strengthening activities to improve posture, balance and trunk stability. Pt. would also benefit from future midline crossing and Ⓑ activities to prepare for future ADL training.

P: Continue OT b.i.d. for 30-minute sessions for 3 weeks for skilled instruction in AROM and strengthening exercises to ↑ trunk stability, balance, and posture. Pt. will demonstrate symmetrical posture in hips and shoulders within 2 weeks in order to sit EOB Ⓘ in preparation for ADL training.

Worksheet 6-3: The Exercise Note

Here are suggestions for the "A" and "P" portions of the note:

A: Pt. demonstrates improved w/c mobility from mod Ⓐ last Thursday to min Ⓐ today. Pt. also demonstrates ↑ AROM in all 5 digits and ↑ activity tolerance in wrist extension (x10) from last Thursday (x5). Pt. would benefit from further strengthening and AROM to reach the 4+ UE strength and 3/4 AROM needed for independence in ADL tasks.

P: Continue Ⓑ UE exercises daily for 1 wk under supervision of a restorative aide to ↑ strength, activity tolerance, and AROM. Skilled OT 3x/wk for work on dressing, bathing, grooming @ 1 hr./visit. Pt. will be Ⓘ in ADLs by discharge in 2 weeks.

(Note by Heather Yamnitz)

Worksheet 6-4: A Treatment Session Devoted to ADL Activities

Write your own "A" and "P" sections for the ADL note.

A: Resident 0x4 and able to make his needs known. Resident able to follow directions if multiple means of communication used. ↓ activity tolerance limits resident's ability to complete ADL tasks. Inability to maintain static postural control creates safety concerns in all ADL tasks. Resident would benefit from NDT to increase stability and postural control as well as continued work on ADL tasks and functional mobility.

P: Resident to be seen 30 minutes b.i.d. for 14 days. Resident will complete ADL tasks of dressing, hygiene, grooming $\bar{c}$ min Ⓓ sitting EOB in 2 weeks.

(Note by Kristen Todd)

Chapter 7

Worksheet 7-1: Evaluating Goal Statements

Which of the following goals has each of the necessary components to be useful in occupational therapy documentation? For each goal that you find to be incomplete or inaccurate in some way, please indicate what it is lacking.

1. By the time of discharge in 2 weeks, patient will be able to dress himself with min Ⓐ for balance using a sock aid and reacher while sitting in a wheelchair.

   This goal has all the necessary components to be useful.

2. Patient will tolerate 10 minutes of treatment daily.

   This goal lacks a function and a time frame. In addition, the behavior (tolerating treatment) is not useful because it is not something a patient needs to do after discharge. This would be better stated as "tolerate 10 minutes of grooming/hygiene activity."

3. Patient will demonstrate increased coping skills in order to live at home with her granddaughter within 2 weeks.

   This goal lacks specificity, and it needs a condition—"coping skills" is far too broad. The coping skills in question need to be specified.

4. Patient will demonstrate 15 minutes of activity tolerance without rest breaks using Ⓑ UE in order to complete ADL tasks before breakfast each morning.

   This goal lacks a time frame, and needs to be turned around to put function first. Patient will be able to complete basic ADL in <15 minutes without rest breaks before breakfast each morning within 2 weeks.

5. In order to be able to toilet Ⓘ self after discharge, patient will demonstrate ability to perform a sliding board transfer w/c ↔ mat within the next week.

   This goal has all the necessary components to be useful, but would be even better if the assist level of the transfer were noted ("i.e., sliding board transfer w/c ↔ mat Ⓘ.")

6. OT will teach lower body dressing using a reacher, dressing stick and sock aid within 3 tx sessions.

   This goal lacks a proper actor and behavior.

7. In order to return to living independently, pt. will demonstrate ability to balance his checkbook.

   This goal lacks a time frame, and would be even better if the assist level for balancing his checkbook were specified (i.e., "ability to balance his checkbook Ⓘ.")

Worksheet 7-2: Writing Realistic, Functional, and Measurable Goals

Without knowing the patient, it is impossible to know what the goal would really be, but here are some suggestions.

Increase Attention Span

Pt. will attend to a cooking activity >10 minutes without having to be redirected within 3 treatment sessions.

Pt. will attend to brushing teeth for >3 minutes c̄ <3 verbal cues by 4/8/02.

Teach the Patient to Follow Directions

In order to increase safety in IADLs within 3 weeks, patient will be able to complete a 3-step task s̄ verbal cues or reminders in 4/5 activities.

By the time of discharge in 2 days, patient will complete 3-step written directions for cooking a packaged meal c̄ min Ⓐ.

Pt. to Dress Upper Body

Pt. will be able to don shirt Ⓘ using the over-the-head method and a button hook within 2 tx sessions.

After skilled instruction, pt. will be able to dress upper body Ⓘ using one-handed techniques and adaptive equipment by 9/15/01.

Increase Endurance

Pt. will perform >10 minutes of continuous standing activity in order to be able bathe her baby by discharge in 1 week.

Within 2 weeks, pt. will complete 30 minutes of Ⓑ UE activity while seated without rest breaks in order to return to her job as a receptionist.

In order to perform light housekeeping tasks, pt. will demonstrate >5 minutes of activity tolerance without rest breaks by discharge on 10/31/01.

Improve Money Management Skills

Pt. will demonstrate ability to make change Ⓘ from $1.00 correctly 3/3 tries within 2 weeks.

Pt. will be able to select ads from the newspaper for an apartment that rents for less than 1/3 of his regular monthly income within the next month.

Decrease Depression

Pt. will spontaneously attend at least three scheduled activities per day by 4/11/01.

Pt. will verbalize an interest in at least one future activity within the next 2 days.

Worksheet 7-3: Mrs. Murphy's Wheelchair Mobility

What is the goal for this patient?

That she will be Ⓘ in w/c mobility by d/c date.

What interventions might you use to help this patient become stronger and learn to propel her wheelchair more successfully?

1. Have her propel her chair to different places.
   - Around her room for grooming and dressing
   - Outside
   - To the gift shop
   - Somewhere she chooses
2. Use backward chaining to help her find her way to a goal location.
3. Mark how far she goes, and ask her to go further each day by passing that mark.
4. Instruct pt. to propel w/c to sink in room to brush hair and clean teeth.
   - Place items needed within her reach.
   - Allow pt. time to figure out what to do, then use verbal cues to guide her through the activity.
5. Instruct pt. to move w/c to other side of the room and back.
   - Use verbal prompts to assist her to avoid running into anything.
   - Use verbal cues to help pt. find handrails and to use both UEs and LEs to propel chair.
   - Have pt. wear shoes.
6. Set up an obstacle course for her with soft things in case she runs into them.
   - Instruct pt. to complete obstacle course without running into anything, and demonstrate where she needs to go.
   - Allow time for pt. to find w/c rails, and use verbal and physical cues to guide her hands if necessary.
   - Allow time for pt. to problem solve on her own before helping her.
   - Use verbal cues if she is unable to maneuver around an obstacle.
7. Put a line on the floor or wall for her to follow.
8. Put things on the wall for her to retrieve.
   - Blue circles to play a game.
   - Family pictures, and have her tell you about each one.
9. Work on upper body strength by having her move items around.
10. Have her gather things in the kitchen or gym and bring them to you.
11. Have her push or pull things out of her way.
12. Take her outside to try the wheelchair on sidewalks and other different surfaces.

Worksheet 7-4: Interrupted Interventions

Rehab Center Setting

1. Set up the task of working on the components of dressing, such as fasteners. For example:
   - Use a button board, or fastener board (such as children use to learn) placed on his lap.

- Place a pajama top on his lap to work on larger buttons.
- Place a pair of pants on his lap to work on handling the zipper pull.
- Place a shoe on his lap to work on tying or fastening the shoe.

2. Set up the task of using adaptive equipment, such as buttonhooks, sock aide, or long shoehorn. For example:
   - Use a buttonhook to unbutton and rebutton the buttons on his shirt.
   - Take off his socks and have him work on getting them back on using the sock aide.
   - Take off his shoes and have him practice using the long shoehorn to don the shoe.
3. Have the patient practice the same compensatory dressing techniques using outer garments such as a sweater or jacket that he can place over his clothes.
4. Have the patient work on the performance components that are limiting his ability to dress. For example:
   - Active range of motion at the shoulder.
   - Fine motor activities for the hand.
   - Activities to increase dynamic balance, if balance is compromised.
   - Sequencing tasks or following directions if cognition is impaired.

Mental Health Setting

1. Interventions relating to self-esteem goals:
   - Join a group working on small craft projects that do not take much skill and can be completed in a short time.
   - Engage him in service projects.
   - Provide opportunities for active listening about his memories, guiding him toward his past successes.
   - Give him small, sincere compliments that he can accept, such as, "Your input during group time was helpful".
   - Ask him to help someone else.
2. Interventions relating to social and leisure skills:
   - Provide opportunities to take part in games (such as cards or checkers) or other activities that require social interaction.
   - Discuss with him his past social and leisure activities to determine his interests.
   - Ask him open-ended questions that require more than a few words to answer.
   - Engage him in the group discussion around the table.
   - Ask him to help another patient do something.

Chapter 8

Worksheet 8-1: Initial Evaluation Report

In each section on the right side of the checklist, make a note of the info found in the preceding initial evaluation.

Background Data

Is the basic demographic data (name, age, sex, date of onset, date of admission, date of referral) present? Note any not present.	All present
Who referred the patient to OT and what services were requested?	Dr. Grantham for evaluation and treatment
Is the patient's medical history and prior level of function included?	Yes
What secondary problems, pre-existing conditions, contraindications, or precautions exist that will impact therapy?	Diabetes
What life stage or environmental factors will impact treatment?	At 68 she would probably be retired
Is the current level of function assessed?	Yes
What do the consumer and her family expect or want from treatment?	Consumer wants to return home; family expectations not recorded

Adapted from Elements of Clinical Documentation *(Revision) (Thomson & Foto, 1995)*

RESULTS OF THE ASSESSMENT

What tests were used? Were there any deviations from the standard procedures?	MME for cognition. Manual muscle test.
What other information or observations were collected besides those from the tests?	Observation of bathing, dressing, toileting, balance, functional mobility.
Are the impairments and their severity identified?	Yes.
Are the functional limitations stated in objective and measurable terms?	Problem #1–Yes. Problem #2–Yes.
What is the rehab potential for this patient?	Good for modified Ⓘ in ADL activities.

Adapted from Elements of Clinical Documentation *(Revision) (Thomson & Foto, 1995)*

TREATMENT PLAN

List one of the functional, measurable long-term goals for this patient.	Pt. will be able to dress with SBA and <3 verbal cues after set-up within 2 weeks.
Are the long-term goals reasonable in relation to the consumer's current status, rehabilitation status, and prior level of functioning?	Yes, with only 2 weeks tx anticipated, priorities have been set. Rehab potential is noted as good for ADLs, but if cognition does not improve it is difficult to tell whether this pt. will be able to return home despite prior level of functioning.
What documentation is there that the patient and family agree with the goals?	None.
Do the short-term goals (objectives) relate to the long-term goals?	Yes.
List one of the short-term goals for problem #2.	Pt. will correctly identify time, date, and situation when asked in 1 week.
Are the interventions that have been selected appropriate to meet the goals?	Yes, but sketchy. More interventions would be good.
What assistive devices are to be used?	Long shoehorn, schedule, list of emergency numbers.
What are the number, frequency, and duration of treatment sessions planned?	10 sessions, 5x wk for 2 weeks.
Are there any recommendations or referrals?	No.

Adapted from Elements of Clinical Documentation *(Revision) (Thomson & Foto, 1995)*

Worksheet 8-2: Progress Notes

Using the following checklist, determine whether the preceding note meets the standard for progress notes.

Criteria	Compliance
What treatment interventions were used?	Instruction in dressing techniques with adaptive equipment and techniques; calendar and schedule posted.
What changes have occurred in this consumer?	Improved dressing skills (dons bra with verbal cues, dons shoes min Ⓐ with long handled shoe horn, don/doff socks mod Ⓐ). Improved orientation to environment. Improved UE strength
What goals have been continued, what goals have been changed, and what goals have been discontinued?	All goals continued.
Have there been any changes in the time frames for reaching goals?	No.
If any assistive devices are being used, how effective are these?	Long handled shoehorn is effective in donning shoes, calendar and schedule are effective in improving orientation.
What contact or conferences have there been with others?	Nursing and others in therapy have been contacted regarding patient's orientation.
Is there a specific plan for the future?	Yes, continue tx.

Adapted from Elements of Clinical Documentation *(Revision) (Thomson & Foto, 1995)*

Worksheet 8-3: Contact, Visit, or Treatment Notes

Using the following checklist, determine whether the note on the preceding page meets the standard for treatment notes.

Criteria	Compliance
What evidence is there of the patient's participation in OT treatment?	Detailed chronological report of the entire treatment session.
What activities, techniques, or modalities were used in this treatment session?	Washed face. Functional mobility supine → sit. Activity tolerance.
If any assistive or adaptive devices were used, is there documentation of whether these were fabricated, sold, or rented, their effectiveness, and what the instructions were for their use?	None noted.
How did this patient (consumer) respond to the treatment provided?	O_2 levels dropped and planned treatment not completed.

Adapted from Elements of Clinical Documentation *(Revision) (Thomson & Foto, 1995)*

Worksheet 8-4: Reevaluation Report

Using the following checklist, determine whether the note on the preceding page meets the standard for evaluation notes.

CRITERIA	COMPLIANCE
What tests were readministered and were the results reported?	Manual muscle test. Grip strength. Palmar and lateral pinch strength. Results documented in note.
How do the current findings compare to the previous results?	Improvement noted.
What are the changes in anticipated functional outcomes?	Anticipate Ⓘ in ADL's with pt. able to return home to live with spouse.
What revisions are being made in the goals, objectives, and interventions?	Goal of min Ⓐ in ADL changed to Ⓘ in ADL.
What revisions are being made in the frequency and duration of treatment?	One additional week requested.

Adapted from Elements of Clinical Documentation *(Revision) (Thomson & Foto, 1995)*

Worksheet 8-5: Discharge Summary #1 (SOAP Format)

Use this worksheet to determine whether thepreceding discharge summary meets the AOTA criteria.

CRITERIA	COMPLIANCE
What interventions were used?	ADL retraining, AROM and strength.
How many treatment sessions were there?	15 of the 20 planned.
How did the consumer respond?	Progress noted.
To what degree were the short- and long-term functional goals achieved?	Partially. This is clearly noted for each activity in the discharge summary.
How does functional status prior to therapy compare to status at discharge?	Clearly noted in the chart.
Is there evidence that a home program was or was not given? Is it attached?	No HEP noted.
What is schedule and specific plan for follow-up?	Plan to see under Medicare B for continued OT.
What are the recommendations pertaining to the consumer's future needs?	Same as above.

Adapted from Elements of Clinical Documentation (Revision) (Thomson & Foto, 1995)

Worksheet 8-6: Discharge Summary #2 (Facility Form)

Use this worksheet to determine whether thepreceding facility discharge summary meets the AOTA criteria.

Criteria	Compliance
What interventions were used?	Adaptive techniques for functional mobility, grooming, hygiene, feeding, dressing, toileting
How many treatment sessions were there?	20
How did the consumer respond?	Met all goals
To what degree were the short- and long-term functional goals achieved?	All met
How does functional status prior to therapy compare to status at discharge?	Status at discharge is improved
Is there evidence that a home program was or was not given? Is it attached?	HEP given and pt. able to perform correctly; HEP was attached
What is schedule and specific plan for follow-up?	PT only
What are the recommendations pertaining to the consumer's future needs?	Adaptive equipment recommended; continue HEP

Adapted from Elements of Clinical Documentation *(Revision)* (AOTA, *2000a*)

Chapter 10

Worksheet 10-1: Soaping Your Note

Indicate beside each of the following statements under which section of the SOAP note you would place it.

__O__ Pt. supine → sit in bed Ⓘ.

__O__ Pt. moved kitchen items from counter to cabinet Ⓘ using Ⓛ hand.

__A__ Problems include decreased coordination, strength, sensation, and proprioception in Ⓛ hand that create safety risks in home management tasks.

__S__ Pt. reports that his fingers are stiff this morning and that he is having trouble handling small items like buttons.

__O__ Pt.'s attention span is <5 minutes.

__A__ Pt's ↑ of 15 minutes in activity tolerance for UE activities permits her to prepare a light meal Ⓘ.

__O__ Child seen in OT clinic to work on fine-motor and visual perceptual skills.

__P__ In order to return to work, pt. will demonstrate an increase of 10 lbs. grasp in Ⓛ hand by 1/3/02.

__A__ Decreased proprioception and motor planning limit patient's ability to dress upper body.

__P__ Continue tx daily for 2 weeks for retrograde massage to Ⓡ hand for edema control

__A__ Patient's correct identification of inappropriate positioning 100% of the time would indicate memory WFL.

__S__ Patient reports that she cannot remember hip precautions.

__A__ Pt. would benefit from further instruction to incorporate total hip precautions into lower body dressing, bathing, and hygiene.

A	Learning was evident by patient's ability to improve with repetition.
O	Pt. does not make eye contact during group session.
A	Pt.'s request to take rest breaks demonstrates knowledge of her limitations in endurance.
O	Pt. wrote bank check for correct amount to pay electric bill with 2 verbal cues.
A	Pt. has progressed to a 3+ muscle grade of extension in Ⓡ wrist extensors this week.
O	Pt. completed weight shifts of trunk x10 in each of anterior, posterior, left and right lateral directions in preparation for standing to perform home management tasks.
O	Pt.'s appearance in mock interview indicates poor judgment and self-concept.

Worksheet 10-2: Subjective

Write a more concise version of this "S."

Pt. reports arthritis in Ⓡ shoulder and knee, pain on weight bearing. During the transfer, pt. requested specific adjustments such as sliding board placement, proximity to bed and approaching transfers from the affected side. Fatigue reported following transfer.

-OR-

Pt. reports significant arthritis in shoulder and knee and prefers to approach transfers from affected side. Pt. reports "It hurts to bear weight on my leg." Pt. also stated w/c → bed sliding board transfers are the most difficult, and reported fatigue after transfer.

-OR-

Pt. reports arthritis in Ⓡ shoulder and knee and pain bearing weight on Ⓡ LE. Pt. able to verbalize needs regarding transfer (placement of board and approach from the affected side). Pt. reports fatigue after transfer.

-OR-

Pt. reports pain in Ⓡ leg when standing due to arthritis in Ⓡ knee & shoulder. Pt. requested re-positioning of sliding board & help to get nearer the bed. Pt. prefers to transfer from affected Ⓡ side and reports fatigue and difficulty during w/c → bed transfer.

-OR-

Pt. reports that transfers continue to be difficult and painful 2° arthritis in Ⓡ shoulder and knee. Pt expressed preference to approach transfer from affected Ⓡ side and expressed fatigue at end of transfer.

Worksheet 10-3: Writing Good Opening Sentences

Rewrite the following opening sentences to show how your skill as an OTA is important in this situation.

1. *Old opening sentence:* Patient seen for morning self-care activities.

   Information found later in the note:

   - Weight bearing precautions raise safety concerns during functional mobility.
   - Hip precautions result in limitations to Ⓘ performance of ADL activities and safe transfers ↔ toilet.
   - Pt. would benefit from skilled instruction in use of adaptive equipment.

   Patient seen in room for skilled instruction on safety strategies and correct use of adaptive equipment during weight bearing activities.

   Patient seen for morning self-care activities to maximize safety and instruct in use of adaptive equipment.

   Patient seen for education on adaptive techniques and equipment for safety in morning self-care activities and functional mobility.

   Patient seen in room for skilled instruction of safety strategies during weight bearing and correct use of adaptive equipment during ADL activities.

2. *Old opening sentence:* Client seen at ACT to work on job skills.

   Information found later in the note:

   - Client demonstrates deficits in sequencing tasks, which ↓ his ability to work Ⓘ.
   - Bilateral coordination problems interfere with client completing an essential job function of opening/closing boxes.

- Sensory registration deficits contribute to client's high distractibility during task completion.

  Client seen at ACT to work on sequencing, bilateral coordination, and sensory registration, which impact his ability to complete work related tasks Ⓘ .

  Client seen at ACT for skilled instruction on task sequencing, Ⓑ coordination, and sensory registration necessary for vocational performance.

  Client seen at ACT for skilled OT to develop compensatory strategies to ↑ sequencing & Ⓑ coordination and sensory registration.

  Client seen for skilled instruction in job sequencing, bilateral integration, and sensori-motor techniques in order to perform work skills Ⓘ .

  Client seen at ACT for task sequencing, ↑ Ⓑ coordination and sensory integration to ↑ work skills.

3. *Old opening sentence:* Client seen for morning dressing.
   Information found later in the note:
   - Deficits include↓ balance and↓ bilateral motor control of upper extremities that↓ ability to safely complete ADL activities and use a manual wheelchair for mobility.
   - Pt. would benefit from skilled education for safety in living at home.

     Pt. would benefit from skilled education for safety in living at home.

     Pt seen in room to work on balance, Ⓑ UE control, and safety in self-care and functional mobility.

     Pt. seen for safety education to↑ balance and Ⓑ motor control of UEs during ADL s and use of w/c @ home.

     Pt. seen to establish strategies which↑ functional balance and↓ fall risk during dressing activities.

     Pt. seen in room to maximize postural stability and ↑ Ⓑ UE motor control while dressing.

     Pt. seen for skilled instruction in safety in performing morning dressing tasks.

4. *Old opening sentence:* Pt. seen in kitchen to work on Ⓘ in cooking.
   Information found later in the note:
   - Patient's problems include decreased dynamic standing balance and inattention of affected UE which raise safety concerns.

     Patient seen in room for skilled instruction in using adaptive equipment and incorporating hip precautions into morning self-care and functional mobility.

     Pt seen in kitchen for positioning and incorporation of affected UE during cooking to↑ safety.

     Pt. seen in OT kitchen to address dynamic standing balance and Ⓛ UE neglect for cooking safety.

     Pt. seen in kitchen for strategies to↑ dynamic standing balance and attention to Ⓛ UE to be safe and Ⓘ during cooking.

     Pt. seen in kitchen to establish strategies for maximizing Ⓘ and safety during cooking.

     Pt. seen in OT kitchen for skilled OT to address dynamic standing balance, inattention to Ⓛ UE, and home safety concerns for Ⓘ in cooking.

Worksheet 10-4: Writing a Complete and Concise "O"—Objective

Consider the following observation of a treatment session. What does it need to make it better?

Toilet transfers:	max Ⓐ
Toileting :	min Ⓐ with SBA 2° inability to support self with Ⓛ arm and to dress
UE dressing :	min Ⓐ , verbal cues, set up, Ⓘ in pulling shirt over head
LE dressing :	min Ⓐ pants to hips
	max Ⓐ pants to waist
	modified Ⓘ don Ⓛ shoe (elastic shoelaces)
	mod Ⓘ to don Ⓡ shoe
Ⓡ hand status:	Ⓡ fingers: small spasticity (index finger greatest amount)
	Thumb: cmc jt. painful in abd. & flex.
	Ⓡ wrist: flaccid

1. An opening line is needed, stating where and why the patient was seen. One possibility would be: *Pt seen bedside for skilled instruction is compensatory dressing techniques.*
2. The categories could be reduced to 3: toileting, dressing, and Ⓡ hand status.
3. It would be helpful to know why the assistance was necessary. Any adaptive techniques or equipment that was used (such as elastic shoelaces) should also be mentioned here.
4. The UE and LE wording should be changed to upper body and lower body because the patient is not dressing only the extremities.

Toileting: Transfers max Ⓐ for balance. Min Ⓐ to support self with Ⓛ UE; max Ⓐ to pull pants up when done.

Dressing: Pt. able to dress upper body p̄ set-up with min Ⓐ for balance when reaching further than arm's length. Pt. Ⓘ in pulling shirt over head. Pt. able to pull pants up to hips with min Ⓐ for balance, but needs max Ⓐ to get pants up to waist using only one hand. Elastic shoelaces allow Ⓘ in donning Ⓛ shoe, but pt. needs mod Ⓐ to get flaccid foot into Ⓡ shoe.

Ⓡ Hand status:
- Ⓡ wrist: flaccid
- Ⓡ fingers: min. spasticity noted
- Ⓡ thumb: painful abduction and flexion at the CMC joint

Worksheet 10-5: Differentiating between Observations and Assessments

Identify which of these statements are assessments and which are observations.

__O__ Pt. is unable to don AFO and shoe Ⓘ for ambulation.

__A__ Patient's inability to don AFO and shoe Ⓘ prevent pt. from ambulating safely around the house to live alone.

__A__ Decreased sensory tolerance limits the patient's attention to task in the classroom.

__O__ Patient requires verbal cues to stay on task due to decreased sensory tolerance.

__O__ Patient was unable to incorporate breathing and energy conservation techniques, requiring several verbal prompts to complete task.

__A__ Inability to incorporate breathing techniques and energy conservation techniques into basic ADL tasks s̄ verbal prompts limits her ability to live alone Ⓘ p̄ discharge.

The following statements are observations of something the OTA saw the patient do. Reword them so that they become assessments.

Patient demonstrated difficulty with laundry and cooking tasks due to memory and sequencing deficits.

A: *Memory and sequencing deficits cause difficulty with home management tasks*

Patient unable to complete homemaking tasks or basic self-care activities independently due to decreased endurance and not following hip precautions.

A: *Patient's decreased endurance and inability to remember hip precautions limit her ability to perform homemaking tasks safely.*

After use of behavior modification techniques, patient displayed courteous behavior for the remainder of the treatment session.

A: *Patient's ability to behave courteously with the aid of behavioral modification techniques indicates good potential for improving problem behaviors in school.*

Worksheet 10-6: Assessment and Plan

Write an assessment and plan for the following patient observation.

O: Patient seen for 30 min. in OT clinic to work on functional movements of Ⓡ UE, dynamic sitting balance, and cognitive skills. Pt. needed mod Ⓐ in shifting weight to get to edge of w/c and max verbal cues to use correct posture and shift feet during standing pivot transfer w/c → mat. Pt. requires max verbal cues to initiate grasp of bag in beanbag activity. Pt. needs mod Ⓐ in reaching with Ⓡ UE. Pt. demonstrated ability to complete Ⓡ UE shoulder flexion required to toss bag approximately 2 feet with max verbal cues. Pt. demonstrated cognitive understanding of activity with mod verbal cues by stating desired goal to be achieved by accurate aim.

Problems/progress

After reading through this note, several problems stood out for this OTA:

- Dynamic sitting balance
- Weight shifting
- Posture
- Transfers
- Decreased AROM in Ⓡ UE
- Cognition

On thinking a little further, she decided that the "cognition" problem might really be one of the following, since he does seem to understand the goal of the activity.

- Short-term memory
- Motor planning
- Problem-solving
- Initiation

Finally the OTA decides that the problem with initiation is probably some combination of problem-solving and motor planning deficit.

Rehab Potential

Ability to Understand the Treatment Goal

The therapist then groups the problems according to the impact they have on the patient's occupational performance. She decides that the first 3 cause difficulty with functional mobility, and are of particular concern because they create safety issues. The motor planning and initiation problem is a concern in the area of self-care, as is the problem with decrease in AROM of the right UE. The fact that he needs continual instruction, whether it is a problem with short term memory or with his ability to problem solve, is likely going to require a lot of attention from a caregiver at home. The patient does, however, understand why he is doing the task she has given him, so as long as the goals are not set too high, he should be able to make good progress in rehabilitation. Her assessment and plan read as follows:

A: Deficits in postural control, dynamic sitting balance, and weight shifting raise safety concerns when transferring. ↓ AROM and motor planning ability negatively impact ability to perform self-care tasks. A need for continual instruction to prevent unsafe performance of ADL tasks requires a high level of caregiver assistance. Patient's ability to understand treatment goal indicates good rehab potential for the goals established. Patient would benefit from continued skilled instruction in activities to ↑ balance, safe functional mobility, and Ⓘ in ADL tasks.

P: Continue tx daily for 3 weeks for skilled instruction in self-care tasks and safe transfers. In 3 weeks patient will be able to transfer safely from wheelchair to bed or toilet c̄ min Ⓐ for balance.

Another OTA might assess the session a little differently. For example:

A: Problems include deficits in motor planning, movement initiation, cognition, and muscle weakness in Ⓡ UE which ↓ safety in ADL tasks and functional mobility. Activity tolerance has improved since last week from <1 minute to >5 minutes without a rest break. Pt. would benefit from skilled OT to increase balance, functional mobility, and grasp/release activities with involved UE in order to ↑ Ⓘ in self-care activities.

P: Continue tx b.i.d. for ½ hour sessions to work on Ⓡ UE movement and cognitive retraining in order to complete grooming activities with min Ⓐ. Pt. will be able to brush teeth with min Ⓐ by the end of 5th tx session.

-OR-

A: Decreased functional use of the Ⓡ UE, decreased sitting balance, and difficulty with sequencing and problem-solving limit ability to perform ADLs. Increased shoulder flexion and motor planning since 12/15/00 and increased understanding of treatment activities indicate good rehab potential. Pt. would benefit from continued skilled OT to increase functional AROM, exercises in grasp, exercises in weight shifting to improve dynamic sitting balance, and evaluation of both cognitive status and ability to initiate activity in order to increase Ⓘ in ADL tasks.

P: Continue b.i.d. for 30-minute sessions for 2 weeks to increase dynamic sitting balance in preparation for ADL training. Pt. will be able to reach for grooming items placed slightly beyond arm's reach without losing balance 3/4 times within 2 weeks.

Worksheet 10-7: The "Almost" Note

What does this note need to make it better?

Here we have a note that seems good on the surface, but demonstrates some problems in critical thinking. The most outstanding problem with this note is that the OTA is mixing her "O" data and her "A" data.

First, there is nothing in the "O" to show that skilled occupational therapy is being provided. The list of observations of assist levels fails to provide the richness of the skill used in treatment. The therapist erroneously puts some of that information in the "A" section, rather than assessing her data.

> *Pt. Ⓘ in dressing while sitting EOB, but is min Ⓐ in dressing when standing with a walker. Ⓛ UE AROM is WFL but Ⓡ UE has deficits noted in shoulder flexion. Pt. SBA in bed mobility when rolling to unaffected side and min Ⓐ in sit → stand 2° to ↓ UE strength. Pt. SBA for transfer to unaffected side in pivot transfer bed → w/c and min Ⓐ w/c → toilet.*

Even in this expanded version, there is nothing to tell us what part of the task the assistance was for. The OTA uses a non-standard abbreviation "VC's". She means verbal cues, but since VC is a standard medical term meaning vital capacity, it is inappropriate in its usage here.

Secondly, the coordination deficits mentioned in the "A" section come out of the blue. There is no mention of coordination in the opening statement "...*for work on dressing and functional mobility*" nor is it mentioned in the "O." Thus the statement that coordination deficits are one of the problems noted and the statement that the patient would benefit from coordination exercises are unsubstantiated. Remember not to introduce any new information in the "A" section of your note.

There is no real assessment of the meaning of the data found in the "S" and the "O." There is a short list of problem areas, but no assessment of their impact of performance areas, and no assessment of the rehab potential shown by the patient's willingness to do "whatever it takes to get out of the hospital."

The best thing for this therapist to do is to rewrite the "O" section, providing a more comprehensive picture of the treatment session. Then she needs to assess her data based on her observations. There needs to be an indication of how the observed data impacts the occupational performance of the patient, before the statements about what the patient would benefit from.

Depending on the assessment she makes, the plan to work on balance may be appropriate, or it may be only one of the things to be addressed.

Worksheet 10-8: Writing Functional and Measurable Goals

Rewrite the following goals in a more logical order, making sure that conditions are present in the goal statement.

1. Pt. will pivot while standing with SBA during toilet transfers in 1 day.

   This goal needs a slight rewording for clarity.

   > *Pt. will be able to perform standing pivot transfer to toilet with SBA within 1 day.*

2. Pt. will be min Ⓐ in dressing UE and LE in 10 days.

   This goal is written in terms of what the patient will be, rather than in terms of what the patient needs. It may seem like a trivial matter, but using the words, "pt. will be min Ⓐ," can indicate a lack of respect for the person receiving treatment. This man is more than an assist level in dressing. It also lacks the conditions under which the patient will dress himself.

   > *Pt. will be able to dress self sitting EOB with min Ⓐ to pull pants over hips in 10 days.*
   >
   > -OR-
   >
   > *Within 10 days, pt. will dress self with min Ⓐ using a dressing stick and long shoehorn.*
   >
   > -OR-
   >
   > *Pt. will dress self with min Ⓐ or balance within 10 days observing 100% of hip precautions.*

3. Pt. will be min Ⓐ in toileting (dressing component) in 3 days.

   This goal would be better if the dressing component were integrated into the main body of the goal, and if the purpose of assistance was stated more clearly.

   Within 3 days, pt. will be able to pull up underpants after toileting with min Ⓐ for balance.

   -OR-

   Within 3 days, pt. will be able to manage clothing after toileting with min Ⓐ to pull pants over hips.

   -OR-

   Pt. will be able to don/doff pants for toileting with min Ⓐ to reach Ⓡ side within 3 days.

   The treatment media also needs to be de-emphasized in writing goal statements.

4. Patient will place 8 ½-inch screws and washers on a block of wood with holes while sitting by 4/10/02.

   Pt. will demonstrate ability to handle small objects needed to return to work by placing eight ½ inch bolts into a block of wood in <5 minutes by 4/10/02.

5. Pt. will make a clock using the appropriate materials while sitting by anticipated discharge on 5/12/02.

   Patient will demonstrate the ability to grasp, place, and release objects of varying sizes needed for IADLs by discharge on 9/3/02.

   -OR-

   Patient will demonstrate ability to follow written instructions of 10 steps by discharge on 9/3/02.

6. Client will stay in his chair without reminders and spend at least 30 minutes lacing the leather billfold during the 45-minute craft group session in 2 weeks.

   This goal is vague and places more emphasis on the media used rather than the performance components involved in the activity.

   Client will attend to task for 30 consecutive minutes during a 45 minute group session without verbal cues.

Worksheet 10-9: Creative Treatment Interventions

Short-term goal: Pt. will spontaneously use the Ⓛ UE as a functional assist for self-care activities at least 3 times in 10 minutes within 4 days.

Interventions: You would want to take Mr. Warren's interests and preferences into account when choosing your treatment interventions. Some of the following are possibilities:

During hygiene activities:

- Instruct him to stabilize the washcloth while putting soap on it.
- Instruct him to hold toothbrush down to apply toothpaste.
- Instruct him to hold a container against his body to open it (toothpaste, deodorant, shaving cream, etc.)

In the kitchen:

- Teach him to make a PBJ sandwich, stabilizing bread with Ⓛ hand, stabilizing peanut butter jar and jelly jar to open them, etc.
- Have him hold a bowl to stir its contents.
- Have him hold a cup to pour powder (such as detergent) into it.
- Teach him to use Ⓡ hand over Ⓛ to wash counter.

During dressing:

- Have him hold shirt while using a buttonhook.
- Show him how to hook thumb into belt loops on Ⓛ side while pulling up Ⓡ side.
- Show him how to hold shoe c̄ Ⓛ UE to put laces in c̄ Ⓡ UE.

Using crafts activities:

- Show him how to hold wood to hammer or screw something into it.
- Help him learn to hold wood to sand it.
- Have him hold copper to tool it.

- Help him make a collage on a topic of interest to him, and stabilize what he is cutting or glueing with the involved UE.
- Have him write by using the Ⓛ UE to stabilize paper to write.

Using cleaning activities:

- In his room, have him clean the mirror, using hand over hand.
- Have him clean golf clubs, stabilizing them with his Ⓛ UE.
- Show him how to wash the car using hand over hand.

Index

Build Your Library

Along with this title, we publish numerous products on a variety of topics. We are sure that you will find the below titles to be an essential addition to your library. Order your copies today or contact us for a copy of our latest catalog for additional product information.

The OTA's Guide to Writing SOAP Notes

Sherry Borcherding, MA, OTR/L and Carol Kappel, MT, OTA

224 pp., Soft Cover, 2002, ISBN 1-55642-551-1, Order #35511, $25.00

The OTA's Guide to Writing SOAP Notes is an instruction manual for teaching a specific skill: documentation as required for reimbursement in occupational therapy. With the current changes in health care, documentation of patient care is essential to meet standards for reimbursement of services. The purpose of this new text is to teach the occupational therapy assistant to write SOAP notes that will be reimbursable under Medicare Part B and managed care. Documentation is learned in the same way that any other skill is learned-instruction and practice. This exceptional, new text offers both the necessary instruction and multiple opportunities to practice, as skills are built on each other in a logical manner.

OTA Study Cards in a Box

Karen Sladyk, PhD, OTR/L, FAOTA, Bay Path College, Longmeadow, MA

208 Study Cards with Carrier, 1999, ISBN 1-55642-394-2, Order #33942, $29.50

OTA *Study Cards in a Box* are 208 review cards dedicated to occupational therapy assistant practice. These review cards are divided into 10 sections designed to provide a general, overall review of important topics in OTA. Topics including patient issues and treatment application are covered, as well as documentation and program management.

These cards are the perfect companion for school, fieldwork, preparation for the certification exam, or occupational therapy practice. The essential information provided on these cards is useful for both the student and clinician. Achieve success with these exciting study tools!

OTA Exam Review Manual

Karen Sladyk, PhD, OTR/L, FAOTA

224 pp., Soft Cover With Disk, 2001, ISBN 1-55642-539-2, Order #35392, $26.95

The OTA *Exam Review Manual* is a holistic study guide that takes the reader from the first day of studying through opening the envelope with the test results. Written specifically for OTA students, this exceptional book incorporates the new domain-focused NBCOT exam and provides simple and complex problem-solving study questions. This exceptional exam review manual includes worksheets, learning assessments, outlines, appendix resources, and web information. Don't wait.... buy this outstanding review manual today!

Contact Us

SLACK Incorporated, Professional Book Division
6900 Grove Road, Thorofare, NJ 08086
1-800-257-8290/1-856-848-1000, Fax: 1-856-853-5991
orders@slackinc.com or www.slackbooks.com

ORDER FORM

Quantity	*Title*	*Order #*	*Price*
	The OTA's Guide to Writing SOAP Notes	35511	$25.00
	OTA Study Cards in a Box	33942	$29.50
	OTA Exam Review Manual	35392	$29.95
		Subtotal	$
		Applicable state and local tax will be added to your purchase	$
		Handling	$4.50
		Total	$

Name: ______________________________
Address: ______________________________
City: ______________ State:______ Zip: ________
Phone:______________ Fax: ______________
Email: ______________________________

- Check enclosed (Payable to SLACK Incorporated): _____
- Charge my: ___ ___ VISA ___ MasterCard

Account #: ______________________________
Exp. date: _______ Signature:______________________

***NOTE:** Prices are subject to change without notice.*
Shipping charges will apply.
Shipping and handling charges are non-returnable.

CODE: 328